International Textbook of Reflective Practice in Nursing

Edited by

Dawn Freshwater, Beverley J Taylor
and Gwen Sherwood

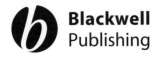

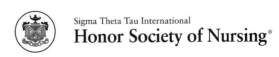

Library of Congress Cataloging-in-Publication Data

International textbook of reflective practice in nursing / editors, Dawn Freshwater,
Beverley J. Taylor, and Gwen Sherwood.
p. ; cm.
Includes bibliographical references and index.
ISBN: 978-1-4051-6051-3 (pbk. : alk. paper)
1. Nursing—Study and teaching. 2. Nursing—Philosophy. I. Freshwater, Dawn.
II. Taylor, Beverley J. (Beverley Joan), 1951– III. Sherwood, Gwen. IV. Sigma
Theta Tau International.
[DNLM: 1. Philosophy, Nursing. 2. Leadership. 3. Nursing, Supervisory.
WY 86 I613 2008]
RT73.I58 2008
610.73—dc22

2007049690

A catalogue record for this book is available from the British Library.

Set in 11/13pt Sabon by Graphicraft Limited, Hong Kong
Printed in Singapore by C.O.S. Printers Pte Ltd

1   2008

Contents

Contributors

Dr Philip Esterhuizen

Philip Esterhuizen PhD, MScN, BA(Cur), DN.Ed, RN is a lecturer in the School of Healthcare, Leeds University. He received his general nursing education in South Africa before specializing in operating room technique. Since then he has specialized in the neurosurgical operating room discipline and neurology before turning to nursing education. He has worked across a variety of settings including acute care, community care and palliative home care; and as a clinical educator, lecturer and researcher. He has worked in different roles in South Africa, the Netherlands, England and Ireland and has provided a series of guest lectures in the United States. Philip's interests include professional socialization, ethics of care, practice and work-based learning and development of professional practice through reflection.

Professor Dawn Freshwater

Dawn Freshwater PhD BA(Hons) RNT RN FRCN is Professor and Dean of the School of Healthcare at Leeds University. She qualified as a nurse 25 years ago and has worked across a number of practitioner, researcher and educational roles during her career to date. She has developed, implemented and evaluated reflective practice and clinical supervision in a variety of global healthcare settings and has authored several books and papers relating to the role of reflection in research and clinical practice. Her work is recognized internationally and has been translated into Hebrew, Chinese, Italian and Russian. Her interests lie in the transformational nature of critical reflection and reflexivity and its potential for mediating between and across disciplines and world views. Dawn, who is also a psychotherapist and counselor, is also editor of the *Journal of Psychiatric and Mental Health Nursing*.

Dr Sara Horton-Deutsch

Sara Horton-Deutsch PhD APRN is an Associate Professor and co-ordinator of the graduate psychiatric/mental health nursing program at Indiana University. This distance-accessible program is based on a reflective-centered framework and Dr Horton-Deutsch facilitates instruction in comprehensive mental health assessment, theory and intervention, and two clinical practicums. Her interests lie in the use of reflective practices as a guide to self-awareness, leadership and interpretive pedagogies. Her research includes the use of mindfulness-based therapeutic interventions in psychiatric/mental health nursing practice.

Professor Gwen Sherwood

Gwen D. Sherwood PhD RN FAAN is Professor and Associate Dean for Academic Affairs at the University of North Carolina at Chapel Hill School of Nursing. Her work focuses on transforming healthcare environments by expanding relational capacity of healthcare providers. She serves Sigma Theta Tau International Honor Society as past chair of the Task Force on the Scholarship of Reflective Practice and currently as Vice President of the Society. Gwen contributes to the profession as past President of the International Association for Human Caring, Chair for the International Network of Doctoral Education Research Interest Group on Work Environments, works globally to advance nursing education and leadership capacity.

Professor Beverley J Taylor

Beverley Taylor PhD MEd RN RM FCN holds the Foundational Chair in Nursing at Southern Cross University, New South Wales, Australia. She is a registered nurse and midwife and has worked in a variety of practice, teaching and research roles over 36 years. Her interests in reflective practice began during her studies in education and she was part of the initiative of introducing reflective practice in nursing to Australia and the world in 1987. Her research is with nurses and midwives using action research and reflection and she is the author of *Reflective Practice: A Guide for Nurses and Midwives*.

Foreword

Like previous works of Dawn Freshwater, she and her distinguished colleagues from around the world have plunged more deeply into the field of reflective practice (RP). This international text delves even more extensively into the already prominent state of the art works by Freshwater and others. This work however, broadens the focus and scope into a multi-faceted lens of application in knowledge-generating discourse that spans clinical scholarship, educational agendas, personal and professional practices as well as leadership. As such this text guides the reader into processes that help to advance nursing as a distinct reflective, discipline and profession of Caring Science, transcending conventional views of nursing-as-doing; rather capturing new aspects of reflection in action.

Freshwater's collection of contributors is renowned and represents the different dimensions of reflective practice from around the globe. Using reflection practice as the core process, this text moves the reader into 'how tos' and processes of *reflection-in-action* that can manifest in creative, innovative and pioneering leadership approaches in research, clinical practice and education.

While extending reflective practice beyond an epistemic focus, *per se*, and beyond conventional clinical agendas, this text simultaneously incorporates evidence and clinical practice demands, yet extends these dynamics into processes which uncover new forms of evidence. Thus, what is revealed is RP as a form of reflective caring – inquiry, a contribution in and of itself. However, the knowledge that is generated through this form of inquiry is a deep authentic form of knowing; capturing inner forms of evidence, highlighting discovery – process as a form of personally and professionally meaningful evidence – grounded from inside-out and outside-in: a new form of empirical knowledge; a new epistemology informed by a reflective ontological starting point as guide and compass throughout. Such discovery becomes enlightened for self and other and in and of itself generates and elevates clinical scholarship, giving voice and active leadership to nursing practice and research.

In the field of education, Freshwater and her capable experienced colleagues point us toward transformative, even therapeutic teaching-learning processes that incorporate and integrate caring and reflection as the essence of nursing. However, the text extends the focus into 'how-to' practices, such as use of reflection for developing curriculum and restoring caring, using reflective narratives, be they in education, practice or research.

This latest work of Freshwater serves as a guide, a resource, and a gift of informed scholarship from around the world. Moreover, it takes us beyond the previous state-of-the-art mindsets – opening new horizons for the emergence of the *art, science and processes* of, and for, reflective practice. Finally this work elevates nursing toward maturity as a distinct human caring-healing contemplative profession and discipline in its own standing.

Jean Watson, PhD, RN, AHN-bc, FAAN
Distinguished Professor of Nursing
Murchinson-Scoville Endowed Chair in
Caring Science
University of Colorado Denver
Anschutz Medical Center
and
Founder/Executive Director
The Watson Caring Science Institute
Boulder, Colorado
February 2008

Acknowledgments

The idea for this book originated from an international working group of the Honor Society of Nursing, Sigma Theta Tau International taskforce on reflective practice. Numerous individuals have contributed to the conceptual and epistemological development of reflective practice as a theorem and as such we cannot do justice to them all in this text, nor can we acknowledge all of our international colleagues who continue to refine and expand both our own and others' ideas and writings. However, we do wish to thank Daniel Pesut for the opportunity to work on the honor society paper on reflective practice and colleagues who supported the development of that paper early on, including Nancy Strijbol and Alma DiCenso. As always we wish to thank Beth Knight and Adam Burbage at Wiley-Blackwell Publishing and Jeff Burnham at the honor society for their support in bringing this text to publication.

Chapter 1

Reflective practice: the state of the art

Dawn Freshwater

Introduction

To title the first chapter of this international text on reflective practice in nursing: 'Reflective practice: the state of the art' has, as you might expect any author to say, been a purposeful, deliberative and mindful choice. However, it is also a humbling and provocative choice of words. The use of the term 'art' is particularly pertinent in the context of reflection in nursing. For many years, nursing has battled with its identity, unsure whether it is an art or a science or indeed both. The literature and indeed the practice of reflection has continuously worked at traversing these two seemingly polar opposites, seeking ways by which both the art and the science, and all that contributes to nursing knowledge, can be articulated and made visible. But of course, as the title also signifies, this is a text that is attempting to capture the current ideologies, opinions, practices (both educational and professional) and research agendas surrounding the expanding and evolving concepts of reflection, critical reflection and reflexivity. A humbling experience indeed. For when one begins to examine the wealth and diversity of data available, it soon becomes apparent that nursing has contributed much to the evolution and application of reflection as a tool for practice improvement, service evaluation, experiential teaching and learning and of course approaches to research. While each chapter in this book stands alone, we have divided the text into three discrete sections, each emphasizing a particular aspect of the whole – knowledge generation, leading and managing practice, that is applications to practice, and the educational imperative of teaching and learning through reflection. In many ways such divisions are arbitrary; nevertheless they also provide a useful structure through which we have been able to retrieve, analyze and synthesize the abundance of data available to us.

This introductory chapter attempts to provide a foundation for the subsequent chapters, in that it illuminates a number of definitions, drawn from a wide range of international sources, referring to and examining the use of terminology in the literature and beginning to prise open the defining features of reflection, critical reflection, reflexivity and associated concepts such as clinical supervision. Later chapters pick up some of the agendas alluded to here, expanding and developing the ideas in order to create a rich tapestry of material for the reader to enjoy, critique, challenge, and feel challenged by, but also importantly to utilize as a tool for stimulating reflection on reflection itself.

Defining the terms

There have been many attempts at defining and pinning down the concept of reflection, spanning over 50 years (if we discount Socrates!), numerous disciplines, authors, poets and artists alike. In fact defining the terms proves challenging for anyone seeking to explicate the nature of reflection, whether the interested reader, or avid and loyal advocate. The intention in this chapter is not to provide a prescriptive and static definition of the concept itself; rather the aim is to make available to the reader a number of perspectives on reflection, both historical and contemporary, by way of positioning the subsequent discussion.

Many of the early attempts at defining reflection drew upon the work of philosophers, one of the earliest being posited by John Dewey (1933: 84) who defined reflection as the 'active, persistent and careful consideration of any belief or supposed form of knowledge in the light of the grounds that support it and the further conclusions to which it tends.' Subsequently several other writers have followed on with their own definitions; nearly always linking reflection to learning from experience. Two decades ago Boyd and Fales (1983) described reflection as an internal learning process in which an issue of concern is examined. Hence, meaning is created and clarified in terms of self, resulting in a changed conceptual perspective. Boyd and Fales (1983) are asserting here that through reflection the individual may come to see the world differently and as a result of new insights can, in turn, come to act differently. Fundamental to this definition is that it involves a change in the self; in other words it is not just individual behavior that has changed but also the individual, hinting at the transformational potential of reflective practice (Freshwater, 1998a, 2000, 2007).

A slightly different interpretation of reflection is offered by (Johns (1995: 24) who over a decade ago defined reflection as 'the practitioner's ability to access, make sense of and learn through work experience, to achieve more desirable, effective and satisfying work.' For Johns the issue of concern is one that Boyd and Fales (1983) allude to, and comes from the experience of conflict or cognitive dissonance in practice. Interestingly, this was also the thrust of the work of Argyris and Schön (1974) who discussed the notion of action theories, positing that all human actions reflect ideas, models or some kind of theoretical notion of purpose and intention and ways in which these purposes and intentions can be executed (Freshwater, 1998a, 1999, 2000; Rolfe *et al.*, 2001). Argyris and Schön (1974) also noted that people often say one thing and do another. Thus, an individual has a personal theory but, when it is operationalized, there is sometimes a contradiction. Based on this idea, they developed the concept of espoused theories (the stated purpose or intention) and theories in use (the attempt to put stated intentions or purpose into action). Hence, espoused theories are those to which individuals claim allegiance; theories in use are those theories which are present when action is executed. Human action therefore is never atheoretical or accidental, even if the theory involved in the action is implicit or tacit. Thus it could be argued that reflection is a way of redeeming theories in use which may be tacit and that practice, in this sense, is theory generating (Freshwater and Avis, 2004; Greenwood, 1998).

Reflection, then, has been and continues to be viewed as a significant learning tool, with Donald Schön (1983) doing much to surface the role of reflection in professional education. Describing the limitations of knowledge derived from technical rationality for practice, Schön (1983: 13) commented on 'the application of research-based knowledge to the solution of instrumental choice that dominates the epistemology of professional practice.' Schön also argued that practitioners have difficulty in utilizing this type of knowledge as it is generated in situations that are context free, thereby ignoring the context of the actual practice situation, drawing attention to the fact that practitioners do not as a rule make decisions based on technical rationality, but on experience. Reflective practice has been developed in nursing as a method of accessing and building upon that experiential (and other types of) knowledge.

Schön identified two main aspects of reflective practice, these being reflection-on-action and reflection-in-action. Nurses and allied health professionals have adopted, adapted, criticized and further developed Schön's thesis and in particular the concepts of reflection in and on action (Burton, 2000; Clouder and Sellars, 2004; Freshwater and Rolfe, 2001; Lahteenmaki, 2005; Rolfe, 1998a). Reflection-on-action is a retrospective process and is the thinking that occurs after an incident with the aim of making sense and using process outcomes to influence future practice. Reflection-in-action relates to the intuitive art of thinking on one's feet. As mentioned, many writers have adopted and developed some of Schön's earlier ideas, linking them to reflexivity, reflection before action and the theory–practice gap, however, his work has also been subject to some heavy criticism since its publication, mainly with regard to the concept of reflection-in-action which, it has been suggested, needs further clarification (Day, 1993; Eraut, 1995). Eraut (1995), for example, made a comprehensive critique of Schön's work, arguing that some of his work was unclear. While Eraut might be justified in pointing out the lack of clarity (and perhaps reflection) in Schön's early works, it should of course be noted that these are Eraut's own reflections, which are also open to further refinement and clarification. Further, from the perspective of a reflective practitioner, all work is work in progress!

In the nursing literature Greenwood (1998) criticized Schön's (1983) model of reflection, arguing that it does not recognize reflection before action; this seems a valid point and one that had been made previously by Reed and Procter (1993) who wrote about the importance of thinking through a particular situation in advance. Burton (2000: 325) notes that this type of reflection before action is 'an essential precursor to introducing clinical supervision,' clearly linking the two concepts (see Chapter 6 for an exploration of the relationship between reflection and clinical supervision). However, it should be noted that this particular view represents a longitudinal view of reflection, based within a linear timeframe drawing upon Western logic, and as such needs to be viewed within that context.

B.J. Taylor (2000: 3), whose writing centers on reflection in nursing practice, defines reflection as

the throwing back of thoughts and memories, in cognitive acts such as thinking, contemplation, meditation and any other form of attentive consideration, in order to make sense of them, and to make contextually appropriate changes if they are required.

This definition, similar to many others, is permissive in that it allows for a wide variety of thinking and types of knowing as the basis for reflection, suggesting that reflective thinking is both a rational and an intuitive process, which potentiates change. Writing of the technical, practical and emancipatory reflection for holistic practice Taylor describes emancipatory reflective practice for overcoming complexities and constraints in holistic healthcare (Taylor, 2003); provides guidance in technical reflection for improving nursing procedures (Taylor, 2002), and on becoming a reflective nurse or midwife, using complementary therapies while practicing holistically (Taylor, 2000).

More recently Freshwater (2002) has linked the practice of reflection to the essential nursing skill of developing self-awareness. Referring to the therapeutic relationship she comments that reflection helps the practitioner to reform their identity through being in relation with themselves, their patients and others, in contrast to having an identity that is formed purely by their surroundings.

According to many theorists reflection has differing levels of depth as well as processes. These levels of reflectivity were discussed in detail by Mezirow (1981, 1990) and although this work is fairly dated in academic terms, it is still viewed as central to the understanding of critical and reflective thinking in both education and health sciences. The levels of reflectivity fall into two broad categories, consciousness and critical consciousness (see Box 1.1).

Mezirow (1981) suggests the idea of a continuum from consciousness to critical consciousness and eventually towards perspective transformation. There are many examples of nurse educationalists and theorists who have adopted Mezirow's (1981) work in their own explorations of reflectivity. Paget (2001), for instance, in his study of practitioners' views of the impact of reflective practice upon clinical outcomes, identified degrees of perspective transformation across a number of practitioners. Freshwater's (2000) research with student nurses also utilized Mezirow's continuum, linking perspective transformation with transformatory learning through clinical supervision.

One of the consequences of having a range of definitions of reflection is that, where reflective practice is concerned, a variety of different frameworks have been generated. Such frameworks provide a useful starting point, as the process of constructing an experience becomes so

---

Box 1.1 Mezirow's (1981) levels of reflectivity.

Consciousness	Critical consciousness
Affective reflectivity	Conceptual reflectivity
Discriminant reflectivity	Psychic reflectivity
Judgmental reflectivity	Theoretical reflectivity

taken for granted that we only become aware that it is a process when it is broken down. However, the availability of many reflective frameworks has, it seems, also added to the confusion and lack of clarity surrounding the concept of reflection itself.

Greenwood (1998) explored this idea in depth, presenting two types of framework existing in relation to the process of reflection, these being single and double loop learning. Generating the concept of single and double loop learning from the work of Argyris and Schön (1974), she notes that the reflective practitioner may respond to a reflection on a situation in two ways. First, the practitioner may search for an alternative means to achieve the same ends; the actions are changed in order to achieve the same outcomes – Greenwood calls this single loop learning. Second, the practitioner may respond not only by exploring alternative means to achieve the intended outcomes, but also examines the appropriateness of the chosen ends. Thus double loop learning 'involves reflection on values and norms and, by implication, the social structures which were instrumental in their development and which render them meaningful' (Greenwood, 1998: 1049).

This could be interpreted to mean that the practitioner is actively engaged in examining themselves and themselves in relation to others, in this instance the social structure within which they operate. This type of reflection requires a great deal of self-monitoring and discipline, but encourages learner autonomy by facilitating in the learner the ability to check their own development (see Chapter 8 for further elucidation on reflection and the therapeutic use of self).

Freshwater (2005, 2007) refers to a similar structure when she notes the distinguishing features of reflection, critical reflection and reflexivity. Simply, she describes reflection as a focussed way of thinking about practice, whatever that practice is. Practices are subject to a degree of scrutiny and examination with the aim of achieving a deeper awareness and understanding of that practice. Critical reflection differs in that the practitioner is not only thinking about their current practices, they are also subjecting the way they are thinking about practice to a degree of interrogation. In other words, the practitioner is thinking about how they are thinking, while simultaneously thinking about their practice. Our ways of thinking have been heavily socialized not only by professional training and academic learning, but also by political, ethical, historical and cultural traditions. As such our thinking is both constructed by our contextual position, and as we exist in that contextual position, we also contribute to constructing it. Having an awareness of this meta-level of contextual influence on both our thinking and our practices and bringing it to bear through reflective processes is termed reflexivity. (Reflexivity is both a method of collecting data about practice and a research method in its own right.) In this sense Freshwater and Rolfe (2001) differentiate reflexivity as a turning back on itself and a type of meta-reflection, emphasizing its critical nature of unsettling previously held assumptions to gain new awareness. This, they argue, is a fundamental purpose of clinical supervision (see Chapter 2 for a detailed explanation of reflexivity).

On reading the literature it would be easy to slip into devising a hierarchy of reflection, as Greenwood (1998) does, putting double loop learning as superior to single loop learning and indeed this could also be an interpretation of Freshwater's (2005a) work. However, this is not useful as it argues for a gap reminiscent of the theory–practice gap in nursing (this is visited again in Chapters 2 and 11). And it might seem obvious to point out, but deep learning can only be made known by coming to the surface. Similarly, reflection and critical reflection are precursors to reflexivity and as such are interdependent. It would seem preferable to advocate an approach to reflection which provides a structure within which structures can be deconstructed. In other words a reflective framework needs to be used flexibly and dynamically. Indeed all work surrounding reflection and its development needs to be relative and evolutionary, paralleling the true nature of reflection (and indeed clinical practice) itself. It could be argued that one such structure is that of clinical supervision, that is to say that clinical supervision could be simply described as a flexible and dynamic structure within which to continuously deconstruct and reconstruct clinical practice.

While outlining the term(s) itself may have caused a few conceptual headaches, it would seem from the literature that it is easier to describe the processes of reflection. However, the continued attempts at defining and refining are essential, for if authors do not share a common definition of reflection, then it is difficult to make comparisons across studies, across geographical boundaries and across disciplines, which in turn makes it difficult to assess the value of reflection in influencing patient outcomes. This may seem at odds with the underpinning philosophy of reflection, which is at base an individual process of learning which reflects individual experience and meaning. It is, by its very nature, localized and there will therefore be some differences in how it is understood and processed and at the same time there will be some shared commonalities which can be transferred across discipline, settings and practices.

Developing expert practice through reflection

The process of reflection

What the literature regarding reflection does have in common is that the complex *process* of reflection is discussed. It is the process of reflection that can be best captured and facilitated in the process of clinical supervision. Most authors identify stages or levels of reflection: Mezirow's (1981) levels of reflectivity have been indicated previously; Schön (1983) identified three levels of reflection, these being reflection, criticism and action; others have also been posited. Atkins and Murphy (1993) in their assessment of the literature discovered that there were three key stages in the reflective process that were shared by most authors. Box 1.2 attempts to synthesize some of these. Several authors have devised reflective cycles to illustrate the integral and circular nature of the reflective process (Gibbs, 1988; Kolb, 1984). It is this reflection as praxis that integrates reflection before action into the reflective process in a non-linear manner involving ongoing development of the practitioner.

Reflection-in-action, it is argued, also involves three distinct but inextricably intertwined processes; McLeod (1996) identifies these as:

- Noticing – a conscious awareness that can be enhanced.
- Reflection – past experiences and understanding, plus the particulars of the present context with the practitioner deeply immersed in the unfolding situation. (Although McCleod (1996) does not refer to reflection-in-action her understanding is described as reflexive, flexible and responsive.)
- Action/Intervening – selecting from a range of options.

The smooth-flowing, tightly bound nature of these components means that while reflection-in-action can be developed, analysis is rarely complete and reflection-on-action is generally required for deeper understanding with the potential for perspective transformation (Taylor *et al.*, 2005). During this dynamic process the practitioner creates a space within which to view their espoused theories, beliefs and values alongside their theories in action with the intent of uncovering contradictions. As the practitioner becomes more aware of their own 'guiding fictions' so the possibility of choice, intentionality and deliberative nursing practice become more of a reality. McLeod (1996: 136) explicates this move to intentional practice succinctly saying that 'the possibility of choice arises from reflexivity, since the person does

---

Box 1.2 The processes of reflection.

First stage   Awareness of uncomfortable feelings and thoughts
                 – experience of surprise
                 – inner discomfort
                 – affective, discriminant, judgmental reflectivity

Second stage Critical analysis of the situation
                 – reflection and criticism
                 – openness to new information and perspectives;
                   resolution
                 – conceptual, psychic and theoretical reflectivity
                 – association, integration, validation and appropriation

Third stage   Development of new perspective
                 – establishing continuity of self with past, present and
                   future; deciding whether and how to take action
                 – perspective transformation
                 – cognitive, affective and behavioral changes
                 – action

---

not respond automatically to events but acts intentionally based on awareness of alternatives.'

As a process, then, reflective practice is multidimensional and seeks to problematize a broad range of professional situations encountered by the practitioner so that they can become potential learning situations (Boyd and Fales, 1983; Burton, 2000; Clouder and Sellars, 2004; Greenwood, 1998; Johns and Freshwater, 1998; Lahteenmaki, 2005; Schön, 1983). Thus reflection enables a continuation of learning and development in which the practitioner grows in and through their practice (Randle, 2002; Todd and Freshwater, 1999). Or as Burton (2000: 326) writes: 'Reflection is a means of formalizing informal learning and development through practice and can be used in the development of the professional portfolio.' Importantly, the practitioner develops an intentionality in regard to practice that has the potential to impact patient care and to refine and define good practice. In this sense, reflective practice should be and is increasingly located as central to practice development, advanced nursing practice and expert practice (Benner, 1984; Burton, 2000; Conway, 1998; Johns, 1998; Johns and Freshwater, 2005; Rolfe, 1998b; Rolfe *et al.*, 2001). While the interpretation of what constitutes an expert practitioner continues to be expanded and refined, it is clear that the practitioner with 'conscious expertise' is one who has a willingness to reflect, is willing to learn from experience, is open minded and does not function in isolation (Dewey, 1933). Interestingly, all that has been said in this previous paragraph about reflective practice has also been reported concerning clinical supervision, almost word for word in some instances. And so the reader may rightly ask: what is the difference between the two? This question is partly answered later in this book (see Chapter 6 specifically), but it is also one that has been rehearsed in the nursing literature several times (Freshwater, 2007).

It is largely agreed that practice development nurses, clinical nurse specialists and nurse consultants act as experts, providing guidance on the development and implementation of best practice, supporting research, innovation and change, and encouraging professional development. Few would disagree that practice development requires that practitioners have opportunities to critically appraise their work (and that of others) in order to ensure that practice is evidence based. To this end many of the advanced practitioners referred to above act as clinical supervisors, facilitating a parallel process to practice development and providing an opportunity for doing the same (see Box 1.3).

Reflective practice can be seen as a companion and precursor to practice development in many ways. Not only does it help to assess whether practice behavior is congruent with espoused values and beliefs, it also assists in the development of autonomy through self-monitoring (Freshwater, 1998b) and accountability through shared learning such as in clinical supervision. Mezirow (1991) considers

---

Box 1.3 Model of reflection for practice development (Freshwater, 2001).

Level of reflection	Methods of reflection	Stages of development
Descriptive	Reflective diaries, reporting incidents Reflection-on-action	Practice becomes conscious
Dialogic	Discourse with peers in various arenas including clinical supervision	Practice becomes deliberative
Critical	Able to provide reasoning for actions by engaging in critical conversation with practice/self/others	Transformation of practice/practice development/ innovation

reflection vital for the building of competence: referring to the process of critical reflection, he contends that questioning the validity of previous learning can lead to a regeneration of knowledge, which in turn produces new or changed meanings. Burton (2000) takes this idea one step further and explicitly links clinical supervision, reflective practice and the development of competence (referring to Benner's framework and that of Blake and Blanchard). In addition it can prevent complacency in everyday practice which, it has been argued, can lead to routinized practice (Walsh and Ford, 1989). As already mentioned effective reflection on practice can lead to more conscious, deliberative and intentional interventions. Furthermore, reflection on beliefs, values and norms offers the opportunity to examine, articulate and generate local philosophies and theories of care, as well as assessing the contribution that individuals make to healthcare delivery at a national level. The generation and assessment of informal theory is something that is inherent in both the process of reflection and in the development of practice.

Models of reflective practice are numerous, just as there is an abundance of models for framing clinical supervision. Models of reflection not only provide a way of redeeming theories in use, emphasizing the importance of theorizing about knowledge grounded in practice, they also represent a dialectic between knowing and doing, regarding practice as a base for knowledge generation (Benner, 1984; Lumby, 1998). Models also enable the practitioner to grasp the purpose of reflective practice, which are sometimes only implied within the specified framework.

Purposes of reflective practice

Argyris and Schön (1974) viewed the purpose of reflective practice as the creation of a world that more faithfully reflects the values and beliefs of people in it, through the construction or revision of people's action theories (Greenwood, 1998). Greenwood (1998: 2) provides a comprehensive summary of the purposes of reflection based on a synthesis of other writers' views. Adapted and updated this is as follows:

- develop individual theories of nursing, to influence practice and generate nursing knowledge (Emden, 1991; Reid, 1993);
- advance theory at a conceptual level to lead to changes at professional, social and political levels (Emden, 1991; Smyth, 1992, 1993);
- facilitate integration of theory and practice (Landeen *et al.*, 1995; McCaugherty, 1991; Wong *et al.*, 1995);

- allow the correction of distortions and errors in beliefs related to discrete activities, and the values and norms which underpin them (Mezirow, 1990);
- encourage a holistic, individualized and flexible approach to care (Freshwater, 2002; Parker, 2002);
- allow the identification, description and resolution of practical problems through deliberative rationalization (Powell, 1989);
- enhance self-esteem through learning (Freshwater, 2000; Johns, 1994, 1995; Randle, 2002);
- heighten the visibility of the therapeutic work of nurses (Freshwater, 2002; Johns, 1994, 1995);
- enable the monitoring of increasing effectiveness over time (Johns, 1995; Landeen *et al.*, 1995);
- enable nurses to explore and come to understand the nature and boundaries of their own role and that of other health professionals (Freshwater, 2002; Johns, 1994, 1995);
- lead to an understanding of the condition under which practitioners practice and, in particular, the barriers that limit practitioners' therapeutic value (Emden, 1991; Johns, 1994, 1995);
- lead to an acceptance of professional responsibility (Johns, 1994, 1995);
- allow a shift in the social control of work. Less direct, overt surveillance over work and much more indirect forms of control through, for example, teamwork, partnerships, collaboration, and so on (Clouder and Sellars, 2004; Gilbert, 2001; Smyth, 1992, 1993);
- provide the opportunity to shift the power to determine what counts as knowledge from an elite, distant from the workplace, to practitioners in the workplace (Freshwater and Rolfe, 2004; Smyth, 1992, 1993);
- allow the generation of a knowledge base that is more comprehensive because it is directly tuned into what practitioners know about practice (Smyth, 1992, 1993); and
- provide the opportunity for a rapid and progressive refocussing of work activity (Smyth, 1992, 1993).

More recent work by Taylor *et al.* (2005) identifies several tangential purposes of reflective practice, including to create spiritual awareness through reflection to address spiritual needs for self and assisting the patient; the development of emotional literacy and emotional intelligence (self-discovery, self-awareness, self-management, motivation and empathy), for self-transformation (Freshwater, 2004) (see Chapter 9); and expand leadership capacity as a transformative change agent (Sherwood and Freshwater, 2005) (see Chapter 7).

In addition Taylor *et al.* (2005) assert that

> *The goal of reflective practice is always in a positive direction, for the growth and discovery of self and one's knowledge, progressing the ability to integrate into one's deepening and expanded practice. In other words, the list of purposes grows as each new venture into reflective practice provides evidence of the usefulness of it, for a wide range of uses in every field of nursing.*

Numerous strategies are identified in the literature to promote the development of reflection, critical reflection and reflexivity. These include journaling, role play, critical incident technique among many others (see Taylor *et al.*, 2005). One such strategy is that of clinical supervision, and it is to this that Chapter 6 is dedicated.

Research and evidence-based practice: reflective strategies

Criticisms of reflective practice mainly center on its failure to demonstrate its usefulness through research studies. Day (1993), for example, points out that how reflection changes practice is unknown. This criticism stems from the argument that the studies which have been carried out relate only to the process of reflection and the practitioner's experience (Hargreaves, 1997). These criticisms are rebuked in the literature as missing the point that the value of reflection is inherent in the experience of the process. As Heath (1998: 291) argues, 'Reflective practice focuses on practice "as it is" and aims to enhance practice from that starting point . . .' The positivist voice is criticized as ignoring the focus of reflective practice as a starting point in favour of a defining point (Heath, 1998).

There is, however, some evidence, albeit minimal, that reflective practice has links with client outcomes. Powell (1989) attempted to access tacit knowledge, often described as defying explanation, using reflection. Powell's (1989) study used Mezirow's levels of reflectivity as signposts to monitor the depth of reflection undertaken by a group of practitioners. Although a small sample was used in this local study, it provides a useful benchmark for development to explore how levels of reflection may enhance practice outcomes. Other studies build upon Powell's (1989) earlier work and indicate that increased depth of reflectivity equates with improved patient care (Freshwater, 1998b). Research studies that have examined the link between reflection and client care include Crandall and Getchell-Reiter (1993), Gray and Forsstrom (1991), Houston (1995), Johns (1998) and McCaugherty (1991).

While skeptics in the literature accept that reflection offers valuable insight into interactions surrounding client care (Tolley, 1995), the main area of contention continues to be about the relatively small gains that are accumulated over time by individual practitioners. It would appear that, to be of value, benefits must be large and rapid with measurable outcomes (Heath, 1998). Unfortunately, the experiential knowledge embedded in everyday practice, and embodied in the subsequent practice narratives, is still judged using scientific measures and is caught in a competitive dialog with empirical knowledge. This does little to progress the development of reflective strategies, as Lumby (1998: 93) points out:

 Reflection as a research tool or method continues to be perceived as questionable as far as issues of validity, reliability and generalization are concerned, often forcing nurses to abandon such strategies or to manipulate them in a way which ensures loss of integrity . . .

resulting in evidence-based practice, reflection and practice development becoming dichotomized and reminiscent of the theory–practice gap.

Newell (1994), it seems, is closer to the mark when he argues, with some vehemence, that reflection needs to be defined in a way which allows its effects on nurses and client care to be tested. This is not only a valid point but allows for individual definitions of reflection to be operationalized in the pursuit of evidence-based practice (see Chapter 3).

In summary, reflection offers a way of accessing deeply embedded personal knowledge. Schön (1983) purports that thinking, via reflection, adds theory to the action while it is occurring, making theory and practice inseparable. Contemporary literature juxtaposes the skills of reflection, the reflective cycle and learning from experience with the skills of clinical supervision.

It would seem then that the state of the art of reflective practice, quite aptly, is in process, is deliberative and like clinical practice is continuously evolving. While the definitions of reflection are flexible and dynamic, mirroring the process of learning from experience, there is some agreement on what the process of reflection involves: namely, an awareness of uncomfortable feelings and thoughts, followed by a critical analysis of feelings and knowledge leading to the development of a new perspective.

The infusion of reflective practice in healthcare demands that awareness and evaluation of self, experience and others is not only a recommended skill but also a requisite of healthcare education, an issue that the literature on experiential learning refers to. Further, in as much as nursing appears to have embraced the concept of reflection, in theory, the literature challenges the practitioner (researcher) to further develop methods of assessing the value of reflective practice in practice.

References

Argyris, C. and Schön, D.A. (1974) *Theory in Practice: Increasing Professional Effectiveness*. Jossey Bass, Washington, DC.

Atkins, S. and Murphy, K. (1993) Reflection: A review of the literature. *Journal of Advanced Nursing*, 18, 1188–92.

Benner, P. (1984) *From Novice to Expert: Uncovering the Knowledge Embedded in Clinical Practice*. Addison-Wesley, Menlo Park, CA.

Boyd, E.M. and Fales, A.W. (1983) Reflective learning key to learning from experience. *Journal of Humanistic Psychology*, 23(2), 99–117.

Burton, A. (2000) Reflection: nursing's practice and education panacea? *Journal of Advanced Nursing*, 31(5), 1009–17.

Clouder, L. and Sellars, J. (2004) Reflective practice and clinical supervision: an interprofessional perspective. *Journal of Advanced Nursing*, 46(3), 262–9.

Conway, J.E. (1998) Evolution of the species 'expert nurse': an examination of the practical knowledge held by expert nurses. *Journal of Clinical Nursing*, 7, 75–82.

Crandall, B. and Getchell-Reiter, K. (1993) Critical decision method: a technique for eliciting concrete assessment indicators from the intuition of NICU nurses. *Advances in Nursing Science, Quality and Cost*, 16(1), 42–51.

Day, C. (1993) Research and the continuing professional development of teachers. An inaugural lecture. University of Nottingham School of Education, Nottingham, UK.

Dewey, J. (1933) *How We Think: A Restatement of the Relation of Reflective Thinking to the Education Process*. Heath, Boston, MA.

Emden, C. (1991) Becoming a reflective practitioner, in Gray, G. and Pratt, R. (eds) *Towards a Discipline of Nursing*. Churchill Livingstone, Melbourne, 335–54.

Eraut, M.E. (1995) Schön shock: a case for reframing reflection-in-action? *Teachers and Teaching*, 1, 9–21.

Freshwater, D. (1998a) The Philosopher's Stone, in Johns, C. and Freshwater, D. (eds) *Transforming Nursing through Reflective Practice*. Blackwell Science, Oxford.

Freshwater, D. (1998b) From acorn to oak tree: a neoplatonic perspective of reflection and caring. *Australian Journal of Holistic Nursing*, 5(2), 14–19.

Freshwater, D. (1999) Communicating with self through caring: the student nurse's experience of reflective practice. *International Journal of Human Caring*, 3(3), 28–33.

Freshwater, D. (2000) Transformatory Learning in Nurse Education. PhD thesis: University of Nottingham, Nottingham, UK.

Freshwater, D. (2001) The role of reflection in practice development. Chapter 4 in Clark, A., Dooher, J. and Fowler, J. (eds) *The Handbook of Practice Development*. Quay Books, Dinton, UK.

Freshwater, D. (ed.) (2002) *Therapeutic Nursing: Improving Patient Care Through Reflection*. Sage, London.

Freshwater, D. (2004) Reflection: A tool for developing clinical leadership. *Reflections on Nursing Leadership*, 2nd quarter, 20–6.

Freshwater, D. (2005) Reflexive Pragmatism, The Natural Harmonic of Caring. 27th International Association for Human Caring, Keynote Address. Lake Tahoe, June 2005.

Freshwater, D. (2007) Reflective practice and clinical supervision: two sides of the same coin? in Bishop, V. (ed.) *Clinical Supervision*, 2nd edn. Palgrave, Basingstoke, UK.

Freshwater, D. and Avis, M. (2004) Analysing interpretation and reinterpreting analysis: exploring the logic of critical reflection. *Nursing Philosophy*, 5, 4–11.

Freshwater, D. and Rolfe, G. (2001) Critical reflexivity: a politically and ethically engaged method for nursing. *NT Research*, 6(1), 526–37.

Freshwater, D. and Rolfe, G. (2004) *Deconstructing Evidence Based Practice*. Taylor & Francis, London.

Gibbs, G. (1988) *Learning by Doing: A Guide to Teaching and Learning Methods*. Further Education Unit, Oxford Polytechnic, Oxford, UK.

Gilbert, T. (2001) Reflective practice and supervision: meticulous rituals of the confessional. *Journal of Advanced Nursing*, 36(2), 199–205.

Gray, J. and Forsstrom, S. (1991) Generating theory from practice: the reflective technique, in Gray, G. and Pratt, R. (eds) *Towards a Discipline of Nursing*. Churchill Livingstone, London.

Greenwood, J. (1998) The role of reflection in single and double loop learning. *Journal of Advanced Nursing Practice*, 27(5), 1048–53.

Hargreaves, J. (1997) Using patients: exploring the ethical dimensions of reflective practice in nurse education. *Journal of Advanced Nursing*, 25(2), 223–8.

Heath, H. (1998) Paradigm, dialogues and dogma: finding a place for research, nursing models and reflective practice. *Journal of Advanced Nursing*, 28(2), 288–94.

Houston, R. (1995) Evaluating quality nursing care through peer review and reflection: the findings of a qualitative study. *International Journal of Nursing Studies*, 32(2), 162–72.

Johns, C. (1994) Nuances of reflection. *Journal of Clinical Nursing*, 3, 71–5.

Johns, C. (1995) Framing learning through reflection within Carper's fundamental ways of knowing in nursing. *Journal of Advanced Nursing*, 22, 226–34.

Johns, C. (1998) Caring through a reflective lens: giving meaning to being a reflective practitioner. *Nursing Inquiry*, 5, 18–24.

Johns, C. and Freshwater, D. (1998) *Transforming Nursing Through Reflective Practice*. Blackwell Science, Oxford.

Johns, C. and Freshwater, D. (2005) *Transforming Nursing through Reflective Practice*, 2nd edn. Blackwell Publishing, Oxford.

Kolb, D. (1984) *Experiential Learning as the Science of Learning and Development*. Prentice Hall, Englewood Cliffs, NJ.

Lahteenmaki, M.-L. (2005) Reflectivity in supervised practice: conventional and transformative approaches to physiotherapy. *Learning in Health and Social Care*, 4(1), 18–28.

Landeen, J., Byrne, D. and Brown, B. (1995) Exploring the lived experiences of psychiatric nursing students through self-reflective journals. *Journal of Advanced Nursing*, 21(5), 878–85.

Lumby, J. (1998) Transforming nursing through reflective practice, in Johns, C. and Freshwater, D. (eds) *Transforming Nursing Through Reflective Practice*. Blackwell Science, London.

McCaugherty, D. (1991) The theory–practice gap in nurse education: its causes and possible solutions. Findings from an action research study. *Journal of Advanced Nursing*, 16, 1055–61.

McLeod, J. (1996) The humanistic paradigm, in Woolfe, R. and Dryden, W. (eds) *Handbook of Counselling Psychology*. Sage, London.

Mezirow, J. (1981) A critical theory of adult learning and education. *Adult Education*, 32, 3–24.

Mezirow, J. (1990) How critical reflection triggers transformative learning, in Mezirow *et al.* (eds) *Fostering Critical Reflection in Adulthood*. Jossey Bass, San Francisco, 1–20.

Mezirow, J. (1991) *Transformative Dimensions of Adult Learning*. Jossey Bass, Oxford.

Newell, R. (1994) Reflection: art, science or pseudo-science. *Nursing Education Today*, 14, 79–81.

Paget, T. (2001) Reflective practice and clinical outcomes: practitioners' views on how reflective practice has influenced their clinical practice. *Journal of Clinical Nursing*, 10, 204–14.

Parker, M. (2002) Aesthetic ways in day-to-day nursing, in Freshwater, D. (ed.) *Therapeutic Nursing*. Sage, London.

Powell, J.H. (1989) The reflective practitioner in nursing. *Journal of Advanced Nursing*, 14(10), 824–32.

Randle, J. (2002) The shaping of moral identity and practice. *Nurse Education in Practice*, 2, 251–6.

Reed, J. and Procter, S. (1993) *Nurse Education: A Reflective Approach*. Edward Arnold, London.

Reid, B. (1993) But we're doing it already! Exploring a response to the concept of reflective practice in order to improve its facilitation. *Nurse Education Today*, 13, 305–9.

Rolfe, G. (1998a) Beyond expertise: reflective and reflexive nursing practice, in Johns, C. and Freshwater, D. (eds) *Transforming Nursing Through Reflective Practice*. Blackwell Science, Oxford.

Rolfe, G. (1998b) The theory–practice gap in nursing: from research-based practice to practitioner-based research. *Journal of Advanced Nursing*, 28(3), 672–9.

Rolfe, G., Freshwater, D. and Jasper, M. (2001) *Critical Reflection for Nurses and the Caring Professions: A User's Guide*. Palgrave, Basingstoke.

Schön, D.A. (1983) *The Reflective Practitioner: How Practitioners Think in Action*. Basic Books, New York.

Sherwood, G. and Freshwater, D. (2005) Doctoral education for transformational leadership in a global context, in Ketefian, S. and McKenna, H. (eds) *Doctoral Education in Nursing: International Perspectives*. Routledge, London.

Smyth, J. (1992) Teachers' work and the politics of reflection. *American Education Research Journal*, 29(2), 267–300.

Smyth, J. (1993) Reflective Practice in Teacher Education and Other Professions. Key Address to the Fifth National Practicum Conference, Macquarie University, Sydney.

Taylor, B.J. (2000) *Reflective Practice: A Guide for Nurses and Midwives*. Allen & Unwin, UK, Melbourne/Open University Press.

Taylor, B.J. (2002) Technical reflection for improving nursing and midwifery procedures using critical thinking in evidence based practice. *Contemporary Nurse*, 13(2–3), 281–7.

Taylor, B.J. (2003) Emancipatory reflective practice for overcoming complexities and constraints in holistic health care. *Sacred Space*, 4(2), 40–5.

Taylor, B., Edwards, P., Holroyd, B., Unwin, A. and Rowley, J. (2005) Assertiveness in nursing practice: an action research and reflection project. *Contemporary Nurse*, 20(2), 324–47.

Todd, G. and Freshwater, D. (1999) Reflective practice and guided discovery: clinical supervision. *British Journal of Nursing*, 8(20), 1383–9.

Tolley, K. (1995) Theory from practice for practice: is this a reality? *Journal of Advanced Nursing*, 21(1), 184–90.

Walsh, M. and Ford, P. (1989) *Nursing Rituals: Research and Rational Actions*. Butterworth-Heinemann, Oxford.

Wong, F., Kember, D., Chung, L. and Yan, L. (1995) Assessing the level of student reflection from reflective journals. *Journal of Advanced Nursing*, 22, 48–57.

Part I

Generating knowledge through reflection

Chapter 2

Reflexivity: using reflection as an approach to research

Beverley J Taylor

Introduction

This chapter describes reflexivity as a tool for researching and improving practice. The relationship between reflection and research is examined, within the contemporary debate around paradigms and paradigm shifts, the search for the 'truth' and evidence-based practice. Responses to the dominant discourse of evidence-based practice are described, showing how reflective practice scholars and researchers have questioned the relegation of qualitative research evidence to the lowest level. Specific research approaches using reflection are described to illustrate ways of finding and validating knowledge in nursing, including: storytelling and narrative; oral history; action research; feminist research and other postmodern approaches.

Reflexivity as a tool for researching and improving practice

Reflexivity is a term used frequently in researching and improving practice, because it alludes to the methods and processes the nurse researcher uses, in order to attain higher levels of awareness and change strategies in relation to the foci of interest. As is the case with many other research terms, reflexivity has been interpreted broadly as it has become more mainstream, especially within qualitative nursing research. Nevertheless, it is important to try to grasp the essential meanings of the term, if it is to be of practical use in discussions about reflective practice and research approaches (Freshwater and Rolfe, 2001).

Research traditions have paid attention to the role of the researcher within the research. For example, in quantitative research, the researcher is directed by controlled methods to create and maintain objectivity within the project, so that the researcher's prejudices, emotions and intentions do not affect data gathering and analysis phases, thereby insuring the validity of the results. This focus on researcher objectivity is discussed later in this chapter, in the section on empirico-analytical research.

In contrast, qualitative research approaches value the subjectivity of researchers as people, who are involved inextricably in the research, yet still able to remain self-aware, thus ensuring that their prejudices, emotions and intentions are not imposed on participants' accounts of their own experiences. As there is a wide objective–subjective chasm between the two research traditions in relation to the role of the researcher within the research, discussions about researcher reflexivity have attempted to shift the paradigm towards proposing different epistemological perspectives, not only about the role of the researcher, but also about the types of knowledge that it is possible to generate and validate within human inquiry.

If we take a starting point, the idea that reflexivity is essentially about the role of the researcher within the research, it is easier to trace the different inflections that have been placed on the term in practice and research literature. For example, Koch and Harrington (1998), influenced by the work of Marcus (1994), identified four forms of reflexivity in relation to ethnography. They suggested that reflexivity could be understood as: being aimed at sustaining objectivity in the empirico-analytical tradition; a means of raising questions about how knowledge is generated and validated through epistemology; from a critical standpoint, in which researchers locate themselves within political and social positions; and from a feminist standpoint, in which researchers embody and perform the politics of the researcher–participant relationship.

Objectivity is the fundamental researcher attitude and orientation within the dominant paradigm of the empirico-analytical tradition. Qualitative nurse researchers applying phenomenological approaches (Hewitt-Taylor, 2002; Rolls and Relf, 2004) influenced by Edmund Husserl (1960) have used bracketing, to lay aside their preconceptions, thereby seeking to sustain levels of objectivity within their projects. Researchers seeking to reduce the potentially distorting effects of their own subjectivity have used reflective journals to 'account for their position and present their rationale in light of this' (Dowling, 2006: 11).

Reflexivity as a means of raising questions about how knowledge is generated and validated through epistemology concerns itself with questions of context. This type of reflexivity explores how a research question is defined to explore an area of interest and the consequences of that definition on knowledge generation and validation processes and outcomes. Epistemological reflexivity is based on the hermeneutics and the writing of Hans Georg Gadamer (1975), who disputed Husserl's objective form of phenomenological reduction, claiming instead that humans are beings in the world through their lived experience; therefore, they cannot separate their Being (ontology) from their knowing (epistemology) interests. The consequences for researchers of this type of reflexivity are that they are involved personally in the research and do not attempt to put their previous assumptions aside, but seek to leave themselves open to what might emerge in the study, so they learn from participants' accounts of their experiences.

Reflexivity from a critical standpoint involves researchers locating themselves within political and social positions, so that they remain mindful of the problematic nature of knowledge and power inherent in human relationships and organizations. Critical standpoint reflexivity draws on the philosophy of Jurgen Habermas (1972, 1973); therefore, researchers critique the socio-political structures in which they are located, reflecting on issues of the effects of power, oppression and disempowerment in hegemonic situations. This form of reflexivity is apparent in research approaches within the qualitative critical paradigm, described later in this chapter.

Reflexivity from a feminist standpoint requires researchers to position themselves within an experiential location, to embody and perform the politics of the researcher–participant relationship, in projects by and for women. Feminist research methods and processes reflect the 'reciprocal nature of the researcher–participant relationship' (Dowling, 2006: 13), examining potential and actual issues of differences in power, while maintaining engaged partnerships with participants.

Even though it is possible to categorize and apply various types of reflexivity, it is not an easy undertaking to achieve involvement without imposition within research projects. For example, Manias and Street (2001) used a critical ethnographic research approach to explore nursing relationships. They acknowledged the difficulties they experienced in recognizing their own taken-for-granted assumptions and values and they were aware of the need to reflect constantly on how these might be surfaced, so they did not impinge on their judgments in the nurses in the study, who had different values to their own. Other researchers have identified difficulties in attaining and maintaining reflexivity, such as the need to identify the difference between being a nurse researcher in a clinical situation, who may feel inclined to offer care (Allen, 2004; Colebourne and Sque, 2004; Whitehead, 2004), in managing their emotional responses to the research participants' accounts (Pateman, 2000; Pellat, 2003; Walsh-Bowers, 2002), and in assessing whether students' reflexivity is authentic (Hargreaves, 2004).

In relation to unraveling the intricacies of reflexivity, if we take as the next point the idea that literature has placed different emphases on a given view of reflexivity, it is reasonable to assume that writers have described the part of the 'elephant' to which they have been oriented. Writers have seen reflexivity as 'the monitored character of the ongoing flow of social life' (Giddens, 1984: 3), and researcher introspection for self-awareness and self-reference (Davies, 1999), thereby emphasizing the interpretive nature of human knowledge. Others have seen reflexivity in a more critical light, emphasizing opportunities for self-appraisal and critique within social contexts (Beck *et al.*, 1994; Hertz, 1997) and 'the examination of the biases, assumptions and values underpinning nursing practice' (Peerson and Yong, 2003: 31). These two positions on reflexivity reflect Taylor *et al.*'s (2006) interpretive and critical categories of qualitative research.

Within and between these interpretive and critical qualitative research positions, authors have described reflexivity variously. Reflexivity is a fundamental method and process in ethnographies and phenomenologies (Koch and Harrington, 1998; Lenny, 2006; Maich *et al.*, 2000; Ross *et al.*, 2005), feminist research (Glass, 2000; King, 1994) and action research (Mantzoukas and Jasper, 2004; Taylor, 2001; Taylor *et al.*, 2002). As these methodologies vary in their emphases of fundamental qualitative research assumptions about knowledge generation, such as giving voice, lived experience, subjectivity and intersubjectivity, context, and the intention to bring about change, they use reflexivity differently to achieve their main intentions and to 'stay true' to key ideas, through maintaining methodological congruency.

Researchers using ethnographic and phenomenological methodologies (Koch and Harrington, 1998; Lenny, 2006; Maich *et al.*, 2000; Ross *et al.*, 2005) define reflexivity as a reflective process for exploring participants' lived experiences and documenting the researcher's role within the project, to prevent the imposition of researcher biases. Feminist researchers (Glass, 2000; King, 1994) see reflexivity as a thoughtful, shared process, bound inextricably in women's experiences, giving them voice and the strategies to identify and transform oppressive situations. Action researchers (Mantzoukas and Jasper, 2004; Taylor, 2001; Taylor *et al.*, 2002) acknowledge the power of reflection using systematic critical questioning to identify and transform problematic social contexts that have previously been accepted as impervious to change.

The researchers within these projects describe various levels of participation, from the involved yet watchful position of participant observer, to being 'one of the others', as a co-researcher. These levels of involvement attempt to reduce the power differences between the researcher and the researched, and increase the participants' sense of ownership of the project. These projects also involve researchers documenting their reflections about their experiences as they participate in the research as participant and researcher within the research context, within multiple levels of researcher involvement. This reflexive transparency intends to reduce the likelihood of imposing researchers' preconceptions on any aspect of the research and to explore the richness of inter-subjective understandings of the research interests, thereby generating knowledge that informs the practice of nursing.

In summary, reflexivity in nursing research has moved beyond the self-indulgent activity of 'navel gazing', to methods and processes that enable researchers to explore, through systematic, critical questioning and appraisal, their roles and influences within projects. Reflexivity in qualitative nursing research projects assumes that human knowledge is subjective and context-dependent and that it is embodied in people's lived experiences. Therefore, qualitative researchers are involved in human-to-human relationships, while remaining vigilant through reflection, to avoid the imposition of their prejudices, emotions and intentions on the conduct and outcomes of research projects. Even so, the involved yet non-imposing position sought by researchers within projects is not easy to attain and maintain, thus researchers need to reflect constantly on their own roles and influences within projects, to bring forward participants' accounts of their experiences.

The relationship between reflection and research

Reflection is fundamental to research, because thinking is fundamental to human life and inquiry. 'Humans have the potential to think and to think about thinking, because we are endowed with the gifts of memory and reflection' (Taylor, 2006: 1). Thinking is used for all kinds of purposes, but the focus highlighted in this chapter is research, because forms of thinking, such as reflecting on experiences, problem

solving, inducing, deducing, synthesizing, interpreting and conceptu-
alizing, are linked inextricably to planning, doing, evaluating and dis-
seminating research.

Reflective practice was defined originally by an educationalist, Donald
Schön, and from its roots in education, reflective practice has been
adopted into nursing. Donald Schön acknowledged the working intelligence of practitioners, and their potential to reflect on and in their
practice, to make sense of their work in a theoretical way, even though
they do not always realize the sophistication of their practical, tacit
knowledge. Schön realized that clinicians need to be taught how to
reflect systematically, so that practice experiences could derive the best
possible outcomes for practitioners and the people they help. When
clinicians are coached to make their knowing-in-action explicit, they
can use this awareness to enliven and change their practice and bridge
the theory–practice gap (Schön, 1983, 1987).

Reflection has been so often defined since Schön's work that it is timely
to return to the original sense of the word. From childhood lessons in
rudimentary physics, we know that in the physical world, reflection
means throwing back from a surface, such as that creating heat, sound
or light (*Australian English Dictionary*, 1999). When the throwing
back occurs, a certain amount of distortion is possible, such as in the
bending phenomenon of refraction when light passes through water.
This is an important fact to remember when considering human
reflection, because reflection may be subject to distorting surfaces and
mediums, to reconstruct the original thoughts and ideas. In connection with human reflection, reflection is

> . . . *the throwing back of thoughts and memories, in cognitive
> acts such as thinking, contemplation, meditation and any other
> form of attentive consideration, in order to make sense of them, and
> to make contextually appropriate changes if they are required.*
> (Taylor, 2006: 2)

This definition is similar to other early representations of reflection
(Argyris and Schön, 1974; Boyd and Fales, 1983; Mezirow, 1981;
Street, 1992) because it is inclusive of many ways of thinking through
rational and intuitive processes, which allow the potential for change.

It is easy to recognize the connections between reflection and research,
especially in terms of ways of thinking and knowing. Humans reflect,
as they review and contrast ideas and construct systematic approaches
to human inquiry. With this fundamental principle in mind, this chapter describes particular ways in which reflection is used in research.

Paradigms and paradigm shifts

In research, a major paradigm shift has been the gradual move to and acceptance of qualitative research, in combination with, or in some cases, in preference to, quantitative research. The main research paradigms and paradigm shifts are the focus of this section.

A paradigm is a broad view or perspective of something. Some people may even say that a paradigm is a 'world view', so it is a comprehensive approach to a particular area of interest. The paradigm of a profession not only concerns the content of the professional knowledge, but also the processes by which that knowledge is produced (Cutcliffe and Goward, 2000; Krasner, 2001a, b; Malinski, 2002). When a paradigm shifts, it shows a movement in thought. For example, humans used to think the world was flat and they were afraid of sailing off the edge, but now we know it is round; having made that paradigm shift, we are content to travel around the planet by sea, land and air.

A paradigmatic view in research provides overall, overarching categories for grouping certain epistemologies. For example, researchers may refer to quantitative or qualitative research. Beyond these modernist classifications lies postmodernism, which resists being represented as a paradigm, even though it has been influential in shifting research paradigms. Postmodern thinking allows researchers to create highly imaginative research strategies to replace the relatively rigid rules and methods that have been reflected in modernist (quantitative and some qualitative) research projects. For example, affirmative postmodern influences encourage researchers to move from their reliance on the 'scientific method' to be guided by their feelings, personal experience, empathy, emotion, intuition, subjective judgment, imagination, creativity and play (Rosenau, 1992). The inclusion of these subjective elements constitutes a major departure from the rules of the 'scientific method' reflected in quantitative research, and constitutes an extension of qualitative researchers' ideas about the role of relative and personal knowledge in their projects.

Even though there has been a paradigm shift towards qualitative research and mixed methods research in nursing and other health professions (Bassett, 2004; Cody, 2000; Streubert-Speziale and Rinaldi-Carpenter, 2003; Young Brockopp and Hastings-Tolsma, 2003), research in the quantitative paradigm still dominates overall, because it attracts major funding from governments and health research sponsors, and it is seen to be more effective in supplying direct, objective facts about the causes, effects and treatment of human illnesses (Courtney, 2005).

Three major categories of research used to generate and verify knowledge in nursing are empirico-analytical, interpretive and critical approaches (Taylor *et al.*, 2006). These categories are reviewed here, to reiterate the idea of paradigms and to highlight the uses of reflection in research.

Empirico-analytical (quantitative) research

Empirico-analytical research is interested in observation and analysis by the scientific method. The scientific method is basically a set of rules for how to do research that can be considered to be rigorous, in the sense that it can be shown to test something over and over again and be consistently accurate (reliability). It also shows that it is testing what it actually intends to test (validity), rather than other things that are there unnoticed (extraneous variables). To achieve this, the scientific method demands that research be as free as possible from the distorting influences of people, such as their ideas, intentions and emotions (subjectivity). In other words, research needs to show that due consideration has been given to achieving objectivity. This process is common to all disciplines that produce scientific knowledge, as it has traditionally been regarded as the best way to build knowledge, through inductive, deductive, theory-building and theory-testing approaches.

Another requirement of the scientific method is that the only research questions that can be asked legitimately are those that can be structured in ways that can be observed and analyzed (by empirico-analytical means) and measured by numbers, percentages and statistics (quantified). This is why research using the scientific method is also referred to as empirico-analytical and/or quantitative research.

Quantitative researchers seek to reduce things of interest to their most focussed and smallest parts (reductionism), in order to study them. They do this based on an underlying assumption that there are cause-and-effect links between certain objects and subjects (variables). It is assumed that these cause-and-effect relationships have a far greater chance of being discovered if the variables in a study are controlled and manipulated carefully. Researchers take a great deal of care to design their projects to insure that they are observing and analyzing the effects of what they intend to study (validity), so that they can demonstrate to 'the scientific community' that the results are significant statistically. This means that they try to confirm or dispute the degree of certainty they can place in cause-and-effect relationships through mathematical explanations.

Health professions have been identified as sciences, because they use the empirical method for their research inquiry. For example, nurses adopted the empirical scientific method because they believed that it was the best way of developing nursing knowledge and of promoting the acceptance of nursing as a valid discipline.

The quantitative research process attempts to find out scientific knowledge by the measurement of elements. This may be at four levels: description, in which elements of a phenomenon are counted; correlations, in which relationships of two or more elements are investigated; explanation, in which one element explains another; and prediction, in which the activity of one element can be predicted from that of another. The quantitative research process uses an empirical method in which data are collected by means of our senses, primarily sight. Many quantitative designs involve testing relationships between phenomena, usually by proposing a hypothesis or statement about the relationship between the variables. Then data are gathered, findings analyzed and conclusions drawn about the findings. This paradigm remains dominant in research, even though there has been a shift towards qualitative and postmodern approaches.

Qualitative research

Qualitative research is interested in questions that involve human consciousness and subjectivity, and value humans and their experiences in the research process. Qualitative research involves finding out about the changing (relative) nature of knowledge, which is seen to be special and centered in the people, place, time and conditions in which it finds itself (unique and context-dependent). Qualitative research uses thinking that starts from the specific instance and moves to the general pattern of combined instances (inductive), so it grows from the ground up to make larger statements about the nature of the thing being explored.

Rather than starting with a statement (hypothesis), qualitative research begins a project with a statement of the area of interest, such as: 'This research will explore the nature and effects of multidisciplinary team relationships in intensive care units.' The measures for ensuring validity in qualitative research involve asking the participants to confirm that the interpretations represent faithfully and clearly what the experience was/is like for them. Reliability is often not an issue in qualitative research, as it is based on the idea that knowledge is relative and is dependent on all of the features of the people, place, time and other circumstances (context) of the setting. People are valued as sources of information and their expressions of their personal awareness (sub-jectivity) are valued as being integral to the meaning that comes out of the research. Rather than saying that something can be claimed as being statistically significant, qualitative research makes no claims to generate knowledge that can be confirmed as certain (absolute).

Given that qualitative research is a vast area, it is easier to think of the paradigm within interpretive and critical categories (Taylor *et al.*, 2006). The main distinction between qualitative interpretive and quali-tative critical research is that interpretive forms are concerned mainly with creating meaning, while critical forms focus on causing socio-political change. All the statements made for qualitative interpretive research apply to critical research, but there is a difference between the two in terms of their intention to bring about social and political change. Qualitative critical research aims overtly to bring about change in the status quo. By working collaboratively with participants as co-researchers to address research problems systematically, qualita-tive researchers within the qualitative critical paradigm work with co-researchers (participants) to identify issues, find solutions and use action strategies to bring about emancipatory socio-political change.

Reflective practice research and evidence-based practice

Nurses identify themselves as professionals, having moved in their practice from occupational to professional status, by attaining the cre-dentials of professionalism, which are: a strong level of commitment; a long and disciplined educational process; a unique body of know-ledge and skill; discretionary authority and judgment; active and cohesive professional organization; and acknowledged social worth and contribution (Freidson, 1970). Tertiary education based on research is integral to professional status. The health profession of medicine has been educated in the tertiary sector much longer than nursing and this is reflected in the strong professional status of doctors as clinicians and the high-priority government support of biomedical research globally into health and illness, especially with the establishment of evidence-based practice.

Evidence-based practice bases current practice on research. Definitions are plentiful for evidence-based practice, including that it is 'the con-scientious, explicit and judicious use of current best evidence in mak-ing decisions about the healthcare of patients' (Sackett *et al.*, 1997: 2) and that it also involves patients' values (Sackett *et al.*, 2000). Dawes (2005: 4) suggests that the simplest definition is that evidence-based practice 'aims to provide the best possible evidence at the point of clinical (or management) contact'. In nursing, French (2002) located more than 14 different definitions of evidence-based practice, with common elements in the definitions of the need for the best evidence, expert clinical decision making, and consideration of patients' needs and values.

Evidence-based practice has been established in medicine for decades and only more recently has evidence-based practice moved its influence into allied health areas. Lockett (1997) traces the development of evidence-based practice to medical researchers in Canada, who wanted to ensure that medical practice was based on research evidence. Sackett *et al.* (1997) attribute the worldwide spread of evidence-based practice to the need for research-based clinical decisions, guidelines and protocols, and the knowledge explosion in new journals in preference to textbook information. The online information format is favored, because it is a quick method of locating up-to-date resources that are often free of cost. Sources of evidence-based practice information are databases (such as Medline, CINAHL, Meditext, PsychINFO, the Digital Theses Programs, Conference Paper Indexes, and library holdings such as the Cochrane Library).

The Cochrane Collaboration based in Oxford, UK, comprises specialized databases of systematic reviews to promote evidence-based practice. These reviews are disseminated through medical journals, CD-ROM, and the internet. There are Cochrane Centers in various countries, including Canada, the UK, the USA and Australia. Evidence-based medicine has grown so rapidly in the UK, Canada and the USA that it is a growth industry that has almost become a medical specialty, with its own journal, *Evidence-Based Medicine*.

The evidence for evidence-based practice is gained systematically by searching for and analyzing research reports accessed though databases and libraries. Pearson and Field (2005: 74) describe the systematic review process as developing the review protocol, asking answerable questions, finding the evidence, appraising the evidence and judging the applicability of the evidence. Appraising the evidence is according to criteria for judging the levels of evidence. Unsurprisingly, quantitative research methods dominate, because of their fit with the generation and validation of biomedical science. Evidence-based practice grew out of the discipline of medicine, therefore it reflects biomedical values about what constitutes knowledge that can be trusted in healthcare.

The almost total absence of qualitative research data as evidence has been a source of critique of evidence-based practice and researchers have attempted to address this deficit. For example, Morse (2003) compiled a comprehensive list of questions as evaluation criteria, relating to relevance, rigor and feasibility, in the sequence of a research proposal. Direct and answerable questions are posed about the research problem or question, investigator capability, and the research methods, context, design, analysis, timelines, budget, subjects, dissemination and outcomes. Other researchers have compiled lists for evaluating qualitative research evidence (Greenhalgh and Taylor, 1997; Horsburg, 2003; Whittemore *et al.*, 2001). The Johanna Briggs Institute in Australia has compiled a hierarchy of four levels of evidence, which is inclusive of qualitative research (Pearson, 2002) and judges the merit of research according to feasibility, appropriateness, meaningfulness and effectiveness. Even so, these alternate qualitative criteria checklists do not change the ratio of quantitative/qualitative methods in levels of evidence, nor do they raise the status generally of qualitative knowledge in the estimation of researchers influenced only by controlled empirico-analytical epistemological methods.

Reflective practice fits well with qualitative research, because they both share key assumptions about the value of the experiencing person within the research project, therefore, lived experience, context and subjectivity are central concepts. This raises a problem for reflective research, if it is to be deemed of value to healthcare, against the levels of evidence that give highest importance to quantitative research methods. In response to the demotion of qualitative research in general and reflective research in particular, authors have critiqued evidence-based practice from various perspectives (Freshwater, 2004; Freshwater and Avis, 2004; Freshwater and Stickley, 2004; Jasper, 2005; Rolfe, 2001, 2003, 2005a, b; Rolfe and Freshwater, 2005).

Taking these responses chronologically, Rolfe (2001: 21) provided a sound foundation for the debate about evidence-based practice and reflective practice research, by arguing that 'reflective practitioners must step outside the dominant paradigm of evidence-based practice in order to reassert the importance of experiential knowledge'. Basing his argument on his experiences, Rolfe (2001: 21) observed that 'it is difficult even to publicly question a mode of practice,' because evidence-based practice has become the catch cry of clinical research, and the act of the writing journal articles dictates an 'academic form' including a literature review and a balanced argument. Boldly persisting against these dominant discourses, Rolfe used a subjective writing style to recount the history of the 'radical origins' of reflective practice, and to align this with the shift of nursing scholarship away from the sole influence of scientific knowledge and technical rationality, towards alternative interpretive and critical paradigms for nursing. Such a paradigm shift was not without its consequences, however, because the 'radical promise of reflective practice . . . became neutralized, as it found itself languishing at the bottom of the hierarchy of nursing evidence' (Rolfe, 2001: 24). He observes correctly that nursing has 'reached a situation, then, where reflection has been divorced from its underpinning philosophy and its emancipatory roots, to the extent that it is forced to justify itself according to the criteria that it formerly rejected' (Rolfe, 2001: 24).

Offering a way through the conundrum of imagining an alternative to technical rationality, Rolfe (2001: 25) proposes principles, through which reflection can 'reclaim its paradigmatic status.' He suggests that: nurses do not judge the reflective paradigm against the technical rational paradigm; we should focus primarily on practice rather than theory; we should value practice, contextual knowledge above theoretical, applied knowledge; practitioners should have a higher status than theorists and researchers; academics should facilitate context-specific practice-based knowledge; pre-registration nurse education should value reflective practice and learning; and greater attention needs to be paid to reflection-in-action, during the event. Taken together, these principles have the potential to invert the present levels of evidence, so that practice-based experience, learning and research become first listed in the reflective paradigm alternative to the evidence-based practice paradigm (Rolfe, 2001: 25–8).

In a response to Newell's (2002) critique of reflection in the nursing curriculum, Rolfe (2003: 7) argued against the 'opinion that reflective practice should be justified by evidence from research, preferably from experimental research methods such as RCTs.' Using the argument that reflective practice and evidence-based practice are both grand theories, with subset methods, processes, techniques and procedures, and that the critical appraisal of evidence-based practice rests on opinion, Rolfe argued that reflective practice should be paid the same respect as evidence-based practice. He summed up his position with the key question: 'If we do not expect to find any research evidence for evidence-based practice, then why do we demand it for reflective practice?'

Freshwater (2004) contributed to the debate about evidence-based practice and other ways of knowing nursing, by viewing the art and science of nursing through a postmodern lens. She argued that 'nursing research is not seen as integral to evidence-based practice' and that 'evidence-based medicine also potentially disregards personal and aesthetic knowledge, what might be termed as indigenous wisdom' (Freshwater, 2004: 8). By reviewing the establishment of levels of evidence-based practice and the low listing of qualitative research methods in that hierarchy, and by contrasting nursing's debate about holism and its relationship to the art of nursing with Carper's (1978) four patterns of knowing in nursing (three of which favour qualitative knowledge), Freshwater directs readers' attention to aesthetics and research in nursing. She suggests that narratives are a source of aesthetic knowing in nursing, and reminds us of Donald's (1998: 24, cited in Freshwater, 2004: 10) remark that 'evidence-based medicine is hardly narrative-free, itself existing within a modern narrative.' In conclusion, Freshwater (2004: 11) encourages 'nurses to continue to lobby for the necessity of qualitative approaches within the evidence-based practice initiative' and to include feedback from consumers, and to draw on aesthetic practices, through qualitative methodologies, 'to facilitate this process.'

Freshwater and Avis (2004) extend the discussion about evidence-based practice and qualitative research to the area of interpretation and analysis. They shift the focus of analysis and interpretation from the rational and creative approach of the hypothetical-deductive testing model to 'a coherent view of knowledge that emphasizes the centrality of dialog with texts, evidence, beliefs and practice' (Freshwater and Avis, 2004: 4). To mount this argument, the authors review the sources of evidence, epistemology and science and the 'lingering influence of positivism,' which succeeds in creating an objective view that continues to impose itself on prescriptive views of knowledge generation and validation. To counter this tendency, Freshwater and Avis (2004: 6) propose a 'pragmatic view of epistemology and the nature of enquiry,' so that 'it is not the means of production of the evidence that constitutes the criterion we use to justify a knowledge claim.'

Reflexivity becomes important in this pragmatic epistemology, because the authors explain that 'understanding achieved through critical reflection is constructed through dialog with the data rather than received from the data' (Freshwater and Avis, 2004: 9). In this view of interpretation and analysis, researchers become responsible for their 'own authority, which demands an awareness of their own discriminatory processes, personal beliefs, and how these originate and are embedded within the broader contexts' (Freshwater and Avis, 2004: 9). Critical reflective awareness is in stark contrast to the dictates of quantitative research approaches, regarded most highly in evidence-based practice.

Freshwater and Stickley (2004: 94) argued that, due to the dominance of evidence-based practice in healthcare and its preference towards rational technical knowledge, 'nursing is becoming more and more technical at the expense of the human qualities of empathy, love and compassion.' In response to this tendency, they make suggestions for a nursing curriculum 'with emotional intelligence at its heart,' such as 'reflective learning experiences,' a 'focus on developing self and dia-logic relationships,' and creative, expressive strategies for developing the human qualities of empathy, self-inquiry and listening (Freshwater and Stickley, 2004: 96).

Other critiques of nursing's tendency to apply uncritically the ramifica-tions of evidence-based practice are the implications it has for the establishment of new nursing roles (Jasper, 2005), the need to be clear conceptually about the sources, importance and effectiveness of levels of evidence (Rolfe, 2005a), and the dismissive responses by evidence-based practice enthusiasts towards thoughtful critiques of the move-ment (Rolfe, 2005b; Rolfe and Freshwater, 2005). Even so, paradigms have the power to resist change. The evidence-based practice and the reflective practice paradigms are 'grand narratives' that propose certain effective qualities in relation to nursing and health practice, but they do not have to be in opposition. Rather, if nurses value difference and continue to critique taken-for-granted positions, they can read between the lines of paradigmatic positions and locate *in between* positions, that take the best of both approaches for the positive progression of nursing practice globally.

Research approaches using reflection

This section describes some research approaches that use reflection as the main or complementary process within their inquiry processes. Many possibilities exist for incorporating reflection in research, includ-ing storytelling and narrative, oral history, action research, feminisms and other postmodern approaches.

Storytelling and narrative

Storytelling and narrative are fundamental to reflective practice and research, because they involve a process of reflecting, to recount and make sense of experiences. The terms 'story,' 'storying,' 'story-telling' and 'narrative' have been used interchangeably (Atkinson, 2002; Graham, 2002; Holloway and Freshwater, 2006; Martin-McDonald, 2003; Walker, 2002). To clarify the matter, Polkinghorne (1988: 18) differentiated a story as a single account reviewing life events in a true or imagined form, and a narrative as a scheme of multiple stories 'that organizes events and human actions into a whole.'

Through research methods, such as conversational interviews and reflective writing, stories can be gathered easily and effectively, as people relate accounts of their experiences. Making sense of the stories can be through a variety of methods to best suit the research questions, aims and objectives. For example, Chan and Schwind (2006) used narrative inquiry (Clandinin and Connelly, 2000) to explore with nurse teachers how they acquired their sense of nursing identity. Some underlying theoretical assumptions of the project were that personal knowledge is significant in people's private and professional lives and that all aspects of 'research, life and learning are intimately related' (Chan and Schwind, 2006: 304).

The researchers recount their own participants' stories 'to explore the common threads . . . while noting the uniqueness of both' (Chan and Schwind, 2006: 305). Through a process of meaning-making, the researchers reread the stories and located threads of their identities as: being cultural and multidimensional; having a sense of belonging; having a tension between uniqueness and conformity; 'living the prescribed identity with a focus on rituals, procedures, systematic process and specialization'; and 'creating a caring learning environment' for nurses as people and students (Chan and Schwind, 2006: 307–10). The researchers concluded that 'understanding how our personal life stories shape our relationships with our patients and students informs our students' continuous learning about the meaning of nursing as a profession' (Chan and Schwind, 2006: 312).

Oral history

Oral history describes the past in a person's own words, which act as raw historical data, to stand alone as a single account, or be validated with other sources, such as historical documents and photographs. Even though oral history has been viewed by some historians as marginal, suspect and trivial (Plummer, 1983) other authors (such as Candida Smith, 2002; Crane, 1997; Tonkin, 1992) promote oral history as a means of 'writing the individual back into collective memory' (Crane, 1997: 1372).

The connections between oral history as a research approach and reflection as a process become apparent immediately, because the person giving the account of her or his life draws actively and systematically on cognitive processes, to enable full descriptions of selected life aspects. For example, Fairman and Mahon (2001: 322) used 15 hours of interviews with Florence Downs to document an oral history. 'Florence Downs is a well-recognized nursing leader, educator, editor, and scholar, who helped shape nursing as an intellectual discipline' and she also wrote extensively on the research–practice nexus. The authors described the first part of Florence's career, from when she first decided to become a nurse, to the early 1970s when she studied towards her doctorate at New York University. From the interviews the researchers

> *gained a sense of how Downs constructed her conceptual universe of nursing, as well as the language and political effectiveness to overcome barriers confronting the intellectual growth of nursing mounted by other nursing leaders as well as traditional academic disciplines* (Fairman and Mahon, 2001: 322).

Reflective topical autobiography incorporates reflection and oral history, so it can be used by people to retrace the events of their lives and the sense they have made of them through reflection. Johnstone (1999: 24) suggests that this form of historical research 'is an important research method in its own right and one which promises to make a substantive contribution to the overall project of advancing nursing inquiry and knowledge.' She explains that ' "re-visioning" of an original topical self-life story demonstrates the enormous creativity of the reflective topical autobiographical method' and

> *leaves open to the self-researcher the opportunity to return at will to his or her life story again to re-read, re-vision and re-tell the story in the light of the new insights, understandings and interpretations of meaning acquired through ongoing lived experience* (p. 25).

Johnstone (1999: 25) cautions that when

> *utilized as a research method, the aim is not to render a 'true' account of the self (as some researchers subscribing to the tenets of positivistic research expect) but to render an account of the lived experience of self that advances shareable understanding of common human experiences.*

Action research

Reflective processes and action research combine well to create effective collaborative qualitative research approaches for identifying and transforming clinical issues, because reflection is a key component of the action research method of planning, assessing, observing and reflecting.

Nursing recognizes the potential of reflective processes to improve practice (Johns, 2003; Stickley and Freshwater, 2002; Thorpe and Barsky, 2001; Taylor, 2000), clinical supervision (Gilbert, 2001; Heath and Freshwater, 2000; Todd and Freshwater, 1999), education (Freshwater, 1999; Johns, 2000; Platzer *et al.*, 2000), and research (Freshwater, 2001; Taylor, 2001; Taylor *et al.*, 2002). Nursing is a complex practice involving knowledge, skills and human connection, so there are many opportunities for using reflection and action research as a collaborative research approach.

The need for social change after World War II created the collaborative research approach of action research (Chein *et al.*, 1948). Kurt Lewin (1946) first used the term 'action research' in the 1940s, when he used a group research process for community projects in postwar America. Lewin's foundational work inspired later versions of action research, including those developed by Australian educationalists such as Carr and Kemmis (1986). The collaborative aspect of action research is that it happens at the site of a concern or practice, and works with the local people as co-researchers, to generate solutions to the problems which they have identified.

Action research involves four phases of collective planning, acting, observing and reflecting (Dick, 1995; Stringer, 1996). Each phase leads to another cycle of action, in which the plan is revised, and further acting, observing and reflecting is undertaken systematically, to work towards solutions to problems. The planning and acting phases may include any appropriate methods of gathering and analyzing data, such as participant observation, reflective journaling, surveys, focus groups and interviews. Cycles of action research lead to further foci and co-researchers can keep an action research approach to their work for as long as they choose, to find solutions to their practice problems.

Nurses have been using action research successfully in a variety of settings with differing thematic concerns (e.g. Keatinge *et al.*, 2000; Koch *et al.*, 2000; Chenoweth and Kilstoff, 1998). Taylor (2001) undertook research to facilitate reflective practice processes in experienced Registered Nurses, in order to: raise critical awareness of practice problems; work systematically through problem-solving processes to uncover constraints; and improve the quality of care given by nurses in light of the identified constraints and possibilities. Twelve experienced female Registered Nurses working in a large Australian rural hospital shared their experiences of nursing during three action research cycles. A thematic concern of dysfunctional nurse–nurse relationships was identified, as evidenced in bullying and horizontal violence. The negotiated action plan was put into place and co-researchers reported varying degrees of success in attempting to improve nurse–nurse relationships. This project confirmed the necessity for reflective practice and continued collaborative research processes in the workplace to bring about a cultural change within nurses' collectives and in the places in which they work which weigh against mutual respect and cooperation in nurse–nurse relationships.

In another project Taylor *et al.* (2002) used a combination of action research and reflective practice processes to explore with six experienced Registered Nurses their tendency towards idealism in their palliative nursing practice, which they defined as the tendency to expect to be 100% effective all of the time in their work. Participants collaborated in generating and evaluating an action plan to recognize and manage the negative effects of idealism in their work expectations and behaviors. Through the reflective processes, participants experienced positive changes in their practice, based on adjusting their responses to their idealistic tendencies towards perfectionism.

Both projects gave nurses a regular forum in which to discuss their reflections on practice and to generate an action plan to bring about change. The benefits of action research and reflection are that there are immediate, practical outcomes for participants, because they can share their experiences with peers, work together on thematic concerns, and bring about local changes in their practice. Thus, co-researchers experience participatory research, while developing their reflective skills, and in this sense the research offers them personal and professional gains in lifelong appreciation for their participation.

Feminist research

Feminism is a social movement concerned with women's issues and lives (Chinn and Wheeler, 1985), and many kinds of feminisms reflect transitions over time in defining and addressing women's concerns, requiring multiple theories to explain the causes of women's oppression (Tong, 1989). Examples of feminisms include liberal, Marxist/socialist, radical, poststructuralist and postmodern representations. Also Glass (2000: 357) described three waves of feminisms and stated emphatically that 'there is no one feminism; feminism is feminisms.'

Even so, feminist researchers agree that 'women are the major focus of feminist research from the beginning to the end of *whole* research projects'; therefore feminist methodology 'concerns research *by* and *for* women . . . putting feminist theory into practice . . . by applying feminist principles directly from feminist premises' (Glass, 2000: 368).

For example, Armishaw and Davis (2002) undertook a critical feminist exploration of women, hepatitis C (HCV) and sexuality. Their beginning assumptions were made explicit, that nurses may exhibit erotophobia and stigmatize patients with HCV. The researchers noted the silence in the literature of women's experiences of living with HCV, thus they decided to explore 'the question of whether living with HCV affected the sexuality of HCV women and if so, in what ways' (Armishaw and Davis, 2002: 194).

The researchers chose a 'modernist feminist paradigm and used critical social theory as a tool that aimed for personal empowerment of the research participants' (Armishaw and Davis, 2002: 196). In congruence with this aim, because 'the very act of speaking and being heard is, in itself, empowering' (p. 196), Judy Armishaw (the honours researcher) collected data via critical conversations and reflective journaling. After institutional ethical clearance, six women, all of whom 'turned out to be' lesbians, were selected using purposive convenience sampling. The women were over 18 years of age, had HCV and had known of their HCV status for over two years.

The audiotaped conversations were listened to over and over again, and transcribed, and the researcher noted that during 'this period of intense familiarity common themes and an overarching analytical framework began to emerge from the data' (p. 197). The framework chosen was Gilligan's (1984) self-in-relations model of moral decision making, because participants spoke of the risks within the dilemma of whether to disclose their HCV status to sexual partners. The themes were 'disclosure,' 'the package,' and 'transcending the package.' 'Disclosure' described the dilemma women experienced in not so much if, but when, to tell their sexual partner of their HCV status. 'The package' referred to the complexity of telling about HCV status in the sense of giving personal information to another and risking being 'boxed' into a stigmatized role, thus enduring being discredited by oneself and others. 'Transcending the package' included 'focusing in the positives of being positive, and having some positive experiences with disclosure' (p. 200).

Other research projects influenced by feminist thought are Anderson and McCann (2002), Boughton (2002), Jackson and Raftos (1997),

Jackson *et al.* (2005), Lumby (1997), Tuttle and Seibold (2002) and Walter *et al.* (1999).

Other postmodern approaches

The postmodern era is providing an eclectic extension to qualitative interpretive and critical research. Postmodernism resists being regarded as a third research paradigm, because postmodern thinking questions many of the taken-for-granted assumptions about knowledge generation and validation in research, and rejects taking on the authority of a 'grand narrative' ('big story' paradigm). Even so, it is possible to discuss postmodern influences on research methods and processes. Postmodernism seeks to upturn cherished notions of the importance of author, text, subject, history, time, theory, truth, representation and politics. It also requires researchers to redefine their basic assumptions, intentions and roles and to make adjustments to their present ways of viewing and doing research and practice (Rosenau, 1992).

The storytelling, oral history, action research and feminism approaches described in the previous section are grand narratives, because they are based on certain assumptions about how knowledge is gained and verified through research methods and processes. The discourse arguing the legitimacy of grand narratives creates various positions. For example, some feminist scholars believe that the emancipatory impulse of feminism is silenced by postmodernism (Benhabib, 1995; Farganis, 1994); therefore, it has no value in advancing the interests of women as members of oppressed groups. In nursing, Kermode and Brown (1995) argued that failure to recognize the grand narratives of capitalism and patriarchy has left uncontested these issues as sources of power. However, there are researchers who have held on to important aspects of a 'grand narrative' while integrating what they see as compatible aspects of postmodernism (Fahy, 1997; Glass and Davis, 1998; Hall, 1999).

Hardin (2003) and Meyer and de Oliveira (2003) have undertaken feminist research influenced by poststructural and postmodern thinking. Hardin was interested in the 'shape-shifting discourses of anorexia nervosa,' particularly 'the circuitous relationship between individuals, the media, and discursive systems' that 'replicate and reinforce the act of self-starvation in young women.' A feminist poststructural methodology was used to expose how 'discourses and institutional practices operate to position young women who take up the subject position of wanting to be diagnosed as anorexic' (Hardin, 2003: 209).

The research was written as a Foucauldian discourse, meaning that anorexia nervosa was the focus not only as an object of interest, but also in the sense of how anorexia is 'constituted by the discourses' in which it emerges. This means that Hardin was interested in examining how anorexia nervosa is created and maintained by shaping agents, such as the media and organizations, so that women become 'types' or 'kinds' of people who starve themselves. After analysis of the messages women posted on online anorexia message boards, Hardin made the point that the media coverage has been so intense as to 'normalize' anorexia nervosa by 'glamorizing' the subject, giving 'anorexics' ways of thinking and acting within the subject position of anorexia nervosa.

Meyer and de Oliveira (2003) are Brazilian researchers who used a poststructural feminist historical-cultural approach to examine breast-feeding policies and the production of motherhood. This research is interesting reading for mothers and midwives, because it provides a strong argument that Brazilian women's bodies have become politi-cized by the government's insistence on promoting the positive aspects of breastfeeding on demand as a woman's responsibility to her child. The researchers made this observation after a discourse analysis of a government document, a breastfeeding promotion guide, which was part of the National Program of Incentive to Breastfeeding (*sic*) (NPIB). The researchers also examined relevant newspaper articles published in Rio Grande do Sul, Brazil, in the year 2000.

Even though many people would claim that breastfeeding is a good thing, the researchers argue that 'there are alternative ways of analyz-ing the issues and consequences of this contemporary emphasis on breastfeeding' (Meyer and de Oliveira, 2003: 11). From this statement the researchers move on to show how medicine and government have represented motherhood. Thus, the best or truest mothers have certain characteristics and functions, against which all other mothers are judged. The researchers argue that the practices of signifying mother-hood involves 'relations of power: the power to name, describe, clas-sify, identify and differentiate' ways of being a mother and a woman, thus including and excluding individuals and groups outside approved social practices (Meyer and de Oliveira, 2003: 12). In other words, good mothers breastfeed on demand and not-so-good mothers do not.

This section provided a snapshot of research projects that have used reflection within their methods and processes. It can be asserted that all qualitative research is implicitly or explicitly reflective in nature, because its basic epistemological assumptions are that knowledge is generated and validated through people's lived experience, as they give personal accounts of their subjective, contextualized experiences. This section described narrative, oral history, action research, feminisms and other postmodern research approaches that use reflection as the main or complementary process within their inquiry processes.

Summary

Reflexivity alludes to the methods and processes the nurse researcher uses, in order to attain higher levels of awareness and change strategies in relation to the foci of interest. Quantitative and qualitative research traditions differ in the ways they have paid attention to the role of the researcher within the research. In quantitative research, the researcher is compelled to create and maintain objectivity within the project, to ensure her or his prejudices, emotions and intentions do not affect data gathering and analyses phases, thereby ensuring the validity of the results. Contrastingly, qualitative research approaches value the subjectivity of researchers as people, involved inextricably in the research, yet able to remain self-aware, thus ensuring that their prejudices, emotions and intentions are not imposed on participants' accounts of their own experiences. Although it is not an easy task to achieve researcher involvement without imposition within research projects, reflexivity in nursing research has moved beyond the self-indulgent activity of 'navel gazing,' to methods and processes that enable researchers to explore, through systematic, critical questioning and appraisal, their roles and influences within projects.

Reflection is fundamental to research, because thinking is fundamental to human life and inquiry. Reflection has been defined and redefined often since Schön's (1983) foundational work, but most definitions are inclusive of many ways of thinking through rational and intuitive processes, which allow the potential for change. The connections between reflection and research are recognized readily, especially in relation to ways of thinking and knowing, because humans reflect, as they review and contrast ideas and construct systematic approaches to human inquiry.

In research, a major paradigm shift has been the gradual move to and acceptance of qualitative research, in combination with, or in some cases, in preference to, quantitative research. When a paradigm shifts, it shows a movement in thought; therefore, a paradigmatic view in research provides overall, overarching categories for grouping certain epistemologies. Beyond the modernist classifications of quantitative or qualitative research lies postmodernism, which resists being represented as a paradigm, even though it has been influential in shifting research paradigms. For example, affirmative postmodern influences encourage researchers to move from their reliance on the 'scientific method' to be guided by their feelings, personal experience, empathy, emotion, intuition, subjective judgment, imagination, creativity and play (Rosenau, 1992). The inclusion of these subjective elements constitutes a major departure from the rules of the 'scientific method' reflected in quantitative research, and constitutes an extension of qualitative researchers' ideas about the role of relative and personal knowledge in their projects.

Three major categories of research used to generate and verify knowledge in nursing are empirico-analytical, interpretive and critical approaches (Taylor *et al.*, 2006). These categories were reviewed in this chapter, to reiterate the idea of paradigms and to highlight the uses of reflection in research.

The health profession of medicine established evidence-based practice, which bases current practice on research. The evidence for evidence-based practice is gained systematically by searching for and analyzing research reports accessed through databases and libraries, and, unsurprisingly, quantitative research methods dominate, because of their fit with biomedical science. This raises a problem for reflective research, if it is to be deemed of value to healthcare, against the levels of evidence that give highest importance to quantitative research methods. In response to the demotion of qualitative research in general and reflective research in particular, authors have critiqued evidence-based practice from various perspectives (Freshwater, 2004; Freshwater and Avis, 2004; Freshwater and Stickley, 2004; Jasper, 2005; Rolfe, 2001, 2003, 2005a, b; Rolfe and Freshwater, 2005).

The concluding section of this chapter described some research approaches that use reflection as the main or complementary process within their inquiry processes. Given that all qualitative research is implicitly or explicitly reflective in nature, because of its basic epistemological assumptions about people's lived experience, subjectivity and contextualized experiences, many opportunities exist for using reflexivity as a research method.

References

Allen, D. (2004) Ethnomethodological insights into insider–outsider relationships in nursing ethnographies of healthcare settings. *Nursing Inquiry*, 11(1), 14–24.

Anderson, J. and McCann, K. (2002) Toward a post-colonial feminist methodology in nursing research: exploring the convergence of post-colonial and black feminist scholarship. *Nurse Researcher*, 9(3), 7–27.

Argyris, C. and Schön, D.A. (1974) *Theory in Practice: Increasing Professional Effectiveness*. Jossey Bass, Washington, DC.

Armishaw, J. and Davis, K. (2002) Women, hepatitis C, and sexuality: a critical feminist exploration. *Contemporary Nurse*, 12(2), 194–203.

Atkinson, R. (2002) The life story interview, in Gubrium, J.F. and Holstein, J.A. (eds) *Handbook of Interview Research: Context and Method*. Sage, Thousand Oaks, CA, 121–40.

Australian Oxford Dictionary (1999) (Moore, B., ed.). Oxford University Press, Oxford.

Bassett, C. (ed.) (2004) *Qualitative Research in Health Care*. Whurr Publishers, London.

Beck, U., Giddens, A. and Lash, S. (1994) *Reflexive Modernisation: Political Traditions and Aesthetics in the Modern Social Order*. Polity Press, Cambridge.

Benhabib, S. (1995) Feminism and postmodernism, in Benhabib, S., Butler, J. Cornell, D. and Fraser, N. (eds) *Feminist Contentions: A Philosophical Exchange*. Routledge, New York.

Boughton, M. (2002) Premature menopause: multiple disruptions between a woman's biological body experience and her lived body. *Journal of Advanced Nursing*, 37(5), 423–30.

Boyd, E.M. and Fales, A.W. (1983) Reflective learning key to learning from experience. *Journal of Humanistic Psychology*, 23(2), 99–117.

Candida Smith, R. (2002) Analytic strategies for oral history interviews, in Gubrium, J.F. and Holstein, J.A. (eds) *Handbook of Interview Research: Context and Method*. Sage, Thousand Oaks, CA, 711–31.

Carper, B. (1978) Fundamental ways of knowing in nursing. *Advances in Nursing Science*, 1(1), 13–23.

Carr, W. and Kemmis, S. (1986) *Becoming Critical: Education, Knowledge and Action Research*. Falmer Press, Lewes, UK.

Chan, E.A. and Schwind, J.K. (2006) Two nurse teachers reflect on acquiring their nursing identity. *Reflective Practice*, 7(3), 303–14.

Chein, I., Cook, S. and Harding, J. (1948) The field of action research. *American Psychology*, 3, 43–50.

Chenoweth, L. and Kilstoff, K. (1998) Facilitating positive changes in community dementia management through participatory action research. *International Journal of Nursing Practice*, 4, 175–88.

Chinn, P.L. and Wheeler, C.E. (1985) Feminism and nursing. *Nursing Outlook*, 33(2), 74–7.

Clandinin, D.J. and Connelly, F.M. (2000) *Teachers as Curriculum Planners*. Jossey-Bass, San Francisco.

Cody, W. (2000) Paradigm shift of paradigm drift? A meditation on commitment and transcendence. *Nursing Science Quarterly*, 13(2), 93–8.

Colebourne, L. and Sque, M. (2004) Split personalities: role conflict between the nurse and the nurse researcher. *NT Research*, 9(4), 297–304.

Courtney, M. (ed.) (2005) *Evidence for Nursing Practice*. Elsevier Churchill Livingstone, Sydney, Australia.

Crane, S. (1997) Writing the individual back into collective memory. *American Historical Review*, 110, 1372–85.

Cutcliffe, J. and Goward, P. (2000) Mental health nurses and qualitative research methods: a mutual attraction? *Journal of Advanced Nursing*, 31(3), 590–8.

Davies, C.A. (1999) *Reflexive Ethnography: A Guide to Researching Selves and Others*. Routledge, London.

Dawes, M. (2005) Evidence-based practice, in Dawes, M., Davies, P., Gray, A., Mant, J., Seers, K. and Snowball, R. (2005) *Evidence-Based Practice: A Primer for Health Care Professionals*, 2nd edn. Elsevier Churchill Livingstone, Edinburgh.

Dick, R. (1995) A beginner's guide to action research. *ARCS Newsletter*, 1(1), 5–9.

Donald, A. (1998) The words we live in, in Greenhalgh, T. and Hurwitz, B. (eds) *Narrative Based Medicine*. BMJ Books, London.

Dowling, M. (2006) Approaches to reflexivity in qualitative research. *Nurse Researcher*, 13(3), 7–21.

Fahy, K. (1997) Postmodern feminist emancipatory research: is it an oxymoron? *Nursing Inquiry*, 4, 27–33.

Fairman, J. and Mahon, M.M. (2001) Oral history of Florence Downs: the early years. *Nursing Research*, 50(5), 322–8.

Farganis, S. (1994) Postmodernism and feminism, in Dickens, D. and Fontana, A. (eds) *Postmodernism and Social Inquiry*. University College Press, London.

Freidson, E. (1970) *Profession of Medicine: A Study of the Sociology of Applied Knowledge*. Harper & Row, New York.

French, P. (2002) What is the evidence on evidence-based nursing? An epistemological concern. *Journal of Advanced Nursing*, 37, 250–7.

Freshwater, D. (1999) Clinical supervision, reflective practice and guided discovery: clinical supervision. *British Journal of Nursing*, 8(20), 1383–9.

Freshwater, D. (2001) Critical reflexivity: a politically and ethically engaged method for nursing. *NT Research*, 6(1), 526–37.

Freshwater, D. (2004) Aesthetics and evidence-based practice in nursing: An oxymoron? *International Journal of Human Caring*, 8(2), 8–12.

Freshwater, D. and Avis, M. (2004) Analysing interpretation and reinterpreting analysis: exploring the logic of critical reflection. *Nursing Philosophy*, 5, 4–11.

Freshwater, D. and Rolfe, G. (2001) Critical reflexivity: a politically and ethically engaged method for nursing. *NT Research*, 6(1), 526–37.

Freshwater, D. and Stickley, T. (2004) The heart of the art: emotional intelligence in nurse education. *Nursing Inquiry*, 11(2), 91–8.

Gadamer, H.-G. (1975) *Truth and Method*, Barden, G. and Cumming, J. (eds). Seabury Press, New York.

Giddens, A. (1984) *The Constitution of Society: Outline of a Theory of Structuration.* University of California Press, Berkeley, CA.

Gilbert, T. (2001) Reflective practice and supervision: meticulous rituals of the confessional. *Journal of Advanced Nursing*, 36(2), 199–205.

Gilligan, C. (1984) *In a Different Voice: Psychological Theory and Women's Development.* Harvard University Press, Cambridge.

Glass, N. (2000) Speaking feminisms and nursing, in Greenwood, J. (ed.) *Nursing Theory in Australia: Development and Application.* Pearson Education Australia, Frenchs Forest, NSW.

Glass, N. and Davis, K. (1998) An emancipatory impulse: a feminist post-modern integrated turning point in nursing research. *Advances in Nursing Science*, 21(1), 43–52.

Graham, I. (2002) Leading the development of nursing within a Nursing Development Unit: the perspectives of leadership by the team leader and a professor of nursing. *International Journal of Nursing Practice*, 9(4), 213–22.

Greenhalgh, T. and Taylor, R. (1997) Papers that go beyond numbers (qualitative research). *British Medical Journal*, 315, 740–3.

Habermas, J. (1972) *Knowledge and Human Interests.* Heinemann, London.

Habermas, J. (1973) *Theory and Practice.* Heinemann, London.

Hall, J. (1999) Marginalization revisited: critical, postmodern, and liberation perspectives. *Advances in Nursing Science*, 22(2), 88–102.

Hardin, P. (2003) Shape-shifting discourses of anorexia nervosa: reconstituting psychopathology. *Nursing Inquiry*, 10(4), 209–17.

Hargreaves, J. (2004) So how do you feel about that? Assessing reflective practice. *Nurse Education Today*, 24, 196–210.

Heath, H. and Freshwater, D. (2000) Clinical supervision as an emancipatory process: avoiding inappropriate intent. *Journal of Advanced Nursing*, 32(5), 1298–306.

Hertz, R. (1997) Introduction, in Hertz, R. (ed.) *Reflexivity and Voice.* Sage, Thousand Oaks, CA.

Hewitt-Taylor, J. (2002) Insider knowledge: issues in insider research. *Nursing Standard*, 16(46), 33–5.

Holloway, I. and Freshwater, D. (2006) *Narrative Research in Nursing.* Blackwell Publishing, Oxford.

Horsburg, D. (2003) Evaluation of qualitative research. *Journal of Clinical Nursing*, 12(2), 307–12.

Husserl, E. (trans.) (1960) *Cartesian Meditations: An Introduction to Phenomenology.* Martinus Nijhoff, The Hague.

Jackson, D. and Raftos, M. (1997) In uncharted waters: confronting the culture of silence in a residential care institution. *International Journal of Nursing Practice*, 3, 34–9.

Jackson, D., Mannix, J., Faga, P. and Gillies, D. (2005) Raising families: urban women's experiences of requiring support. *Contemporary Nurse*, 18(1–2), 97–107.

Jasper, M. (2005) Editorial. New nursing roles – implications for nursing. *Journal of Nursing Management*, 13, 93–6.

Johns, C. (2000) Working with Alice: a reflection. *Complementary Therapies in Nursing and Midwifery*, 6, 199–303.

Johns, C. (2003) Easing into the light. *International Journal for Human Caring*, 7(1), 49–55.

Johns, P.R. (2000) *Becoming a Reflective Practitioner*. Blackwell Science, London.

Johnstone, M.-J. (1999) Reflective topical autobiography: an underutilized interpretive research method in nursing. *Collegian*, 6(1), 24–9.

Keatinge, D., Scarfe, C., Bellchambers, H., McGee, J., Oakham, R., Probert, C., Stewart, L. and Stokes, J. (2000) The manifestation and nursing management of agitation in institutionalized residents with dementia. *International Journal of Nursing Practice*, 6, 16–25.

Kermode, S. and Brown, C. (1995) Where have all the flowers gone: nursing's escape from the radical critique. *Contemporary Nurse*, 4(1), 8–15.

King, K. (1994) Method and methodology in feminist research: what is the difference? *Journal of Advanced Nursing*, 20(1), 19–22.

Koch, T. and Harrington, A. (1998) Reconceptualizing rigour: the case for reflexivity. *Journal of Advanced Nursing*, 28(4), 882–90.

Koch, T., Kralik, D. and Kelly, S. (2000) We just don't talk about it: men living with urinary incontinence and multiple sclerosis. *International Journal of Nursing Practice*, 6, 253–60.

Krasner, D. (2001a) Qualitative research: a different paradigm – Part 1. *Journal of Wound, Ostomy and Continence Nursing*, 28(2), 70–2.

Krasner, D. (2001b) Qualitative research: a different paradigm – Part 2. *Journal of Wound, Ostomy and Continence Nursing*, 28(3), 122–4.

Lenny, M.J. (2006) Inclusion, projections of difference and reflective practice: an interactionist perspective. *Reflective Practice*, 7(2), 181–92.

Lewin, K. (1946) Action research and minority issues. *Journal of Social Issues*, 2, 34–46.

Lockett, T. (1997) Traces of evidence. *Healthcare Today*, July/August, 16.

Lumby, J. (1997) Liver transplantation: the death/life paradox. *International Journal of Nursing Practice*, 3, 231–8.

Maich, N.M., Brown, B. and Royle, J. (2000) 'Becoming' through reflection and professional portfolios: the voice of growth in nursing. *Reflective Practice*, 1(3), 309–24.

Malinski, V. (2002) Research issues: nursing research and the human sciences. *Nursing Science Quarterly*, 15(1), 14–20.

Manias, E. and Street, A. (2001) Rethinking ethnography: reconstructing nursing relationships. *Journal of Advanced Nursing*, 33(2), 234–42.

Mantzoukas, S. and Jasper, M. (2004) Reflective practice and daily ward reality: a covert power game. *Issues in Clinical Nursing*, 13, 925–33.

Marcus, G.E. (1994) What comes (just) after 'post'? The case of ethnography, in Denzin, N. and Lincoln, Y. (eds) *Handbook of Qualitative Research*. Sage, London.

Martin-McDonald, K. (2003) Being dialysis-dependent: a qualitative perspective. *Collegian*, 10(2), 29–33.

Meyer, D. and de Oliveira, D. (2003) Breastfeeding policies and the production of motherhood: a historical-cultural approach. *Nursing Inquiry*, 10(1), 11–18.

Mezirow, J. (1981) A critical theory of adult learning and education. *Adult Education*, 32, 3–24.

Morse, J.M. (2003) A review committee's guide for evaluating qualitative proposals. *Qualitative Health Research*, 13, 833–51.

Newell, R. (2002) Commentary: Is there a place for reflection in the nursing curriculum? *Clinical Effectiveness in Nursing*, 6, 42–3.

Pateman, B. (2000) Feminist research or humanistic research? Experiences of studying prostatectomy. *Journal of Clinical Nursing*, 9(2), 310–16.

Pearson, A. (2002) Nursing takes the lead: redefining what counts as evidence in Australian healthcare. *Reflections on Nursing Leadership*, 4th quarter, 18–21.

Pearson, A. and Field, J. (2005) The systematic review process, in Courtney, M. (ed.) *Evidence for Nursing Practice*. Elsevier Churchill Livingstone, Sydney, Australia.

Peerson, A. and Yong, V. (2003) Reflexivity in nursing: Where is the patient? Where is the nurse? *The Australian Journal of Holistic Nursing*, 10(1), 30–45.

Pellat, G. (2003) Ethnography and reflexivity: emotions and feelings in fieldwork *Nurse Researcher*, 19(3), 28–37.

Platzer, H., Blake, D. and Ashford, D. (2000) Barriers to learning from reflection: a study of the use of groupwork with post-registration nurses. *Journal of Advanced Nursing*, 31(5), 1001–8.

Plummer, K. (1983) *Documents of Life: An Introduction to the Problems and Literature of a Humanistic Method*. George Allen & Unwin, London.

Polkinghorne, D.E. (1988) *Narrative Knowing and the Human Sciences*. State University of New York, Albany, NY.

Rolfe, G. (2001) Reflective practice: Where now? *Nurse Education in Practice*, 2, 21–9.

Rolfe, G. (2003) Is there a place for reflection in the nursing curriculum? A reply to Newell. *Clinical Effectiveness in Nursing*, 7(1), 61.

Rolfe, G. (2005a) Editorial. Evidence-based practice and the need for conceptual clarity. *Practice Development in Health Care*, 4(1), 1–2.

Rolfe, G. (2005b) Response. Where is John Paley when you need him? *Nursing Philosophy*, 6, 152–5.

Rolfe, G. and Freshwater, D. (2005) 'To save the honour of thinking': a slightly petulant response to Griffiths. *International Journal of Nursing Studies*, 42, 363–9.

Rolls, L. and Relf, M. (2004) 'Bracketing Interviews': A Method for Increasing Objectivity in Bereavement and Pallitiave Care Research. Paper presented at Methodology of Research in Palliative Care. Third research forum of the EAPC, Stresa, Italy.

Rosenau, P. (1992) *Post-Modernism and the Social Sciences: Insights, Inroads and Intrusions*. Princeton University Press, Princeton, NJ.

Ross, A., King, N. and Firth, J. (2005) Interprofessional relationships and collaborative working: encouraging reflective practice. *Online Journal of Issues in Nursing*, 10(1), 12p.

Sackett, D.L., Richardson, W.S., Rosenbery, W. and Haynes, R.B. (1997) *Evidence-Based Medicine: How to Practice and Teach EBM*. Churchill Livingstone, New York.

Sackett, D.L., Straus, S.E. and Richardson, W.S. (2000) *Evidence-Based Medicine: How to Practice and Teach EBM*, 2nd edn. Churchill Livingstone, New York.

Schön, D.A. (1983) *The Reflective Practitioner: How Practitioners Think in Action*. Basic Books, New York.

Schön, D.A. (1987) *Educating the Reflective Practitioner*. Jossey-Bass, London.

Stickley, T. and Freshwater, D. (2002) The art of loving and the therapeutic relationship. *Nursing Inquiry*, 9(4), 250–6.

Street, A. (1992) *Inside Nursing: A Critical Ethnography of Clinical Nursing*. State University of New York, Albany, NY.

Streubert-Speziale, H. and Rinaldi-Carpenter, D. (2003) *Qualitative Research in Nursing: Advancing the Humanistic Perspective*. Lippincott, Philadelphia, PA.

Stringer, E. (1996) *Action Research: A Handbook for Practitioners*. Sage, Thousand Oaks, CA.

Taylor, B. (2000) *Being Human: Ordinariness in Nursing* (adapted and reprinted). Southern Cross University Press, Lismore, NSW, Australia.

Taylor, B.J. (2001) Identifying and transforming dysfunctional nurse–nurse relationships through reflective practice and action research. *International Journal of Nursing Practice*, 7(6), 406–13.

Taylor, B.J. (2006) *Reflective Practice: A Guide for Nurses and Midwives*, 2nd edn. Open University Press, Milton Keynes, UK.

Taylor, B.J., Bulmer, B., Hill, L., Luxford, C., McFarlane, J. and Stirling, K. (2002) Exploring idealism in palliative nursing care through reflective practice and action research. *International Journal of Palliative Nursing*, 8(7), 324–30.

Taylor, B., Kermode, S. and Roberts, K. (2006) *Research in Nursing and Health Care: Evidence for Practice*, 3rd edn. Thomson, Australia.

Thorpe, K. and Barsky, J. (2001) Healing through self-reflection. *Journal of Advanced Nursing*, 35(5), 760–8.

Todd, G. and Freshwater, D. (1999) Reflective practice and guided discovery: clinical supervision. *British Journal of Nursing*, 8(20), 1383–9.

Tong, R. (1989) *Feminist Thought: A Comprehensive Introduction*. Unwin Hyman, Sydney, Australia.

Tonkin, E. (1992) *Narrating Our Pasts: The Social Construction of Oral History*. Cambridge University Press, Cambridge.

Tuttle, L. and Seibold, C. (2002) Ethical issues arising when planning and commencing a research study with chemically dependent pregnant women. *Australian Journal of Advanced Nursing*, 20(4), 30–6.

Walker, A. (2002) Safety and comfort work of nurses glimpsed through patient narratives. *International Journal of Nursing Practice*, 8(1), 42–8.

Walsh-Bowers, R. (2002) Constructing qualitative knowledge in psychology: students and faculty negotiate the social context of inquiry. *Canadian Psychology*, 43(4), 163–78.

Walter, R., Davis, K. and Glass, N. (1999) Discovery of self: exploring, interconnecting and integrating self (concept) and nursing. *Collegian*, 6(2), 12–15.

Whitehead, L. (2004) Enhancing the quality of hermeneutic research: decision trail. *Journal of Advanced Nursing*, 45(5), 512–18.

Whittemore, R., Chase, S. and Mandle, C. (2001) Validity in qualitative research. *Qualitative Health Research*, 11, 522–37.

Young Brockopp, D. and Hastings-Tolsma, M. (2003) *Fundamentals of Nursing Research*, 3rd edn. Jones & Bartlett, Boston, MA.

Chapter 3

Developing an evidence-based approach to clinical practice

Dawn Freshwater

Introduction

In Chapter 2 we described approaches to research and outlined the nature of paradigmatic debates in relation to reflection and reflection practice. As we explained, nursing practice has traditionally been viewed through a scientific lens, relying upon a medical model which has been and continues to be firmly rooted in the scientific method and philosophy. Thus the professional knowledge that has driven nursing practice has, in the main and until fairly recently, been derived from a model of technical rationality that has dominated the thinking about professions and has shaped professional practice (Freshwater and Broughton, 2000). Even definitions of nursing have derived their origins from medicine with nurses being socialized into the position of having little or no voice (Johns and Hardy, 1998) (see Chapter 10 for further discussions on the nature of nursing). A wealth of literature is available to suggest that nurses experience themselves as dominated by the medical profession (Brunning and Huffington, 1985; Capra, 1982; Friedson, 1970). This has never been more debated than most recently with the introduction of the evidence-based practice movement. In this chapter the concepts of reflection and evidence-based practice are examined in tandem, and importantly complementary processes and discrepancies are identified. It is argued that reflective practice and in particular critical reflection and reflexivity provide systematic and deliberative ways in which to improve and develop clinical practice.

Context

Reflexivity is an important concept, not only in critical science to ensure that the object of critical intent is as far as possible critically appraised, but also in the carrying out of action research and reflective practice. The idea of reflexivity, which was clearly defined in Chapter 2 and is raised at various points throughout this text, was central to the development of George Kelly's personal construct theory (1955).

Kelly (1955) posits that in the process of reflexivity we become our own personal scientists (see also Chapter 8 on the therapeutic use of self). In 1998 Rolfe illuminated a similar process in nursing through the work of Benner (1984) and Schön (1983). The reflexive practitioner, argues Rolfe (1998), is able to modify their practice on the spot, responding to their hypothesis testing. This cycle of continuous conscious reflection-in-action is recognized both in education and the research process. Examples include Kolb's (1984) experiential learning cycle, Pfeiffer and Jones' (1980) learning cycle and Poincaré (1952) and Wallas' (1926; cited in Neville, 1989) stages of learning, all of which follow a similar pattern.

The development of nursing theory and the acknowledgment of the differing sources of knowledge brought to a head the argument that nursing theory and nursing practice must be founded on a scientific basis (Akinsanya, 1985; Freshwater, 2000; Salvage, 1998). The phrase 'evidence based' has increasingly entered the discourse around effectiveness in nursing and has captured the attention of both managers and researchers alike – the former because of its seeming potential to rationalize costs in healthcare provision, the latter because of its association with the problems related to the lack of adoption of research findings in nursing. However, evidence-based practice is not just about ensuring that practice is substantiated by research, it is also concerned with accountable practice and as such requires that the practitioner makes their private knowledge public. Translating research into practice, thereby ensuring that nursing care is founded upon the best available evidence, is certainly a challenge for the profession, not least in achieving this from a stance of professional accountability and responsibility.

That nursing ought to be founded on a scientific basis is not a new proposition. Chater in 1975, for example, not only maintained that nursing should be underpinned by scientific principles but added that patient care should be founded on defensible research-based findings. Dramatic changes in healthcare and the rapid growth of care pathways and integrated care delivery systems have focussed practitioners' attention on enhancing patient outcomes through providing effective nursing practice. It could be argued that not to base nursing practice on research is unethical; however, overcoming the barriers to the application, dissemination and uptake of research findings that continue to plague the world of nursing is not an easy task. Clearly nursing practice should be based on the best available evidence, and it is fair to say that there are now more opportunities for developing and increasing nursing research than ever before; however, nursing care and treatment remains largely unaffected by research findings.

In order to facilitate the utilization of research findings and to ensure that nursing practice is founded on the best available evidence, the nursing professional has been assigned the task of implementing evidence-based practice. Evidence-based practice demands that nurses maintain a closer compatibility between their nursing beliefs and their nursing care.

Research was briefly attended to in Chapter 2, and as it is not the main focus of this book it will not be revisited in any depth here. Suffice it to say that, whatever the approach, the researcher is an extremely important component of any research effort and the purposes, intentions and goals of the researcher will contribute significantly to the design, process and outcome of the research study. In some of the more contemporary approaches to the research design there is a democratization of the research endeavor. The researcher's status is not privileged over the participants, who may be referred to as co-researchers/ investigators. This fits well with the recent trend towards consumer involvement in research, which emphasizes active involvement of consumers in the research process, rather than the use of consumers as the 'subjects' of research.

In order for nurses to develop a healthier attitude towards research and evidence-based practice a strong infrastructure needs to be in place, one that provides significant experience not only of developing clinical guidelines but also of fostering local adaptation to increase ownership of relevant research findings prior to addressing the practical problems of time and workload constraints. The benefits, rewards and reinforcements that nurses receive for utilizing research-based knowledge in practice need to be made explicit through increased institutional support.

Cultural barriers relate to the lack of preparation that practitioners receive for research in clinical practice. In the new healthcare environment practitioners must learn systematic review of research literature, critical appraisal of research findings and synthesis of empirical evidence with contextually relevant experience, that is clinical experience and opinion-based processes. Practitioners often 'do' research as part of an academic course which can provide some theoretical grounding in methods of searching and appraising research. Once back in practice, knowledge and experience gained is not always followed through; in other words, results are rarely disseminated to colleagues, published locally and nationally, re-evaluated in the context of a developing clinical environment and presented at local research forums. In addition research that is undertaken as part of an educational course tends to focus on the course requirements rather than influencing local practice through researching local, regional and national initiatives – such findings are not deemed relevant to practice and are not utilized (Bishop and Freshwater, 2004). A further barrier is the process of gaining ethical approval for research projects, a lengthy and sometimes medicalized process which can feel obstructive to nurses interested in pursuing clinical research. Thus, whilst many nurses are aware of the importance of research findings, they are rarely applied; this is not surprising given the level of preparation practitioners are afforded, for even published findings require the skills of interpretation and translation for effective transference to the practitioner's own context and client group.

Quality of evidence is assessed in terms of its level, knowledge gained through systematic review and randomized controlled trials being viewed as the most robust evidence. Many nurses do not feel comfortable with the idea of randomized controlled trials (RCTs) in nursing which do not always capture knowledge based in esthetic experience and personal knowledge such as intuition. Therein lies a tension between nursing research and the current interpretation of evidence-based practice as indicated in the hierarchy of evidence.

There are those who argue that knowledge is contingent and that research questions emerge after a period of familiarity within a specific setting and that as such practitioners are best placed to ask research questions (Fox, 1999; Freshwater and Rolfe, 2001, 2004). Hence research questions should be developed in such a way that the theoretical consequences will be of direct practical relevance with the appropriate methodology employed to operationalize the research question. One final point on barriers relates to the lack of understanding of the differences between research and audit and their inherent processes. There continues to be a level of confusion amongst clinical nurses, and indeed some researchers and auditors, as to the similarities and differences between audit and research (Close and Cheater, 1996). This chapter does not seek to detail the differences but it is worth noting that there is a distinct difference between the two although both have links with quality and ensuring good practice.

Evidence-based practice

As has already been discussed, the literature surrounding evidence-based practice originates in medicine and implies a strong orientation towards randomized controlled trials, with 'best evidence' being synonymous with empirical research or scientific evidence (French, 1999; Sackett *et al.*, 1996). There are many definitions of evidence-based practice, evidence-based healthcare, evidence-based nursing and the forerunner of them all – evidence-based medicine, some of them more 'user friendly' than others. Sackett *et al.* (1996) talk about 'conscientious, explicit and judicious use of current best evidence'; Hicks (1997) includes 'due weight accorded to all valid relevant information' in his definition of evidence-based healthcare and 'using contemporaneous research findings' is part of Rosenberg and Donald's (1995) definition of evidence-based medicine.

It is said that the purpose of evidence-based medicine is to 'base medical decisions on the best available evidence' (Sackett and Rosenberg, 1995). Best *medical* practice has long been determined by the use of randomized controlled trials and as such evidence-based *nursing* practice is a by-product of the modernist-rationalistic paradigm, the dominant paradigm of the medical profession. The current paradigm shift that is taking place throughout the Western world in science means that rationalistic, positivistic science is no longer the dominant worldview. Nursing is not a linear process and, whilst the nursing process has attempted (unsuccessfully, we might argue) to order decision making in nursing, it cannot order the world of the patient, which is non-linear, acausal and often chaotic (Marks-Maran, 1999). Nursing decisions are often made in random intuitive ways based, it would seem, on personal opinion, professional expertise and interpretation of the immediate context. Hence nursing must find an understanding of evidence-based practice that is congruent with its own philosophies and beliefs and that fits with the emerging paradigm shift (Marks-Maran, 1999).

Evidence-based practice is reached by following a number of steps. Rosenberg and Donald (1995) suggest:

- formulating a clear clinical question from a patient's problem;
- searching the literature for relevant clinical articles;

- evaluating (critical appraisal) the evidence for its validity and usefulness;
- implementing useful findings in practice.

Rosswurm and Larrabee (1999) also devised their own tried and tested model for evidence-based practice, based upon theoretical and research literature. The model follows six stages:

(1) Assess the need for change in practice.
(2) Link problem interventions and outcomes.
(3) Synthesize best evidence.
(4) Design practice change.
(5) Implement and evaluate change in practice.
(6) Integrate and maintain change in practice.

The overall success of the model is dependent upon the level of meticulousness maintained at each of the six stages. Whilst most practitioners are easily able to identify and assess the need for change in practice (the first stage in this model), the subsequent five stages of the model may pose more of a challenge. Further, not all clinical problems are amenable to research (White, 1997) and it is not often that a single problem arises with a single appropriate intervention.

Research, evidence-based practice and clinical governance

Several national and international initiatives have been developed to facilitate the implementation of evidence-based practice. The National Institute for Clinical Excellence (NICE), the Clinical Standards Advisory Board (CSAG) and the Committee for Health Improvement in England along with Health Service Frameworks (HSR) are amongst those tasked with ensuring that clinical practice is underpinned by a substantive body of evidence. Similarly, international policies reflect the drive towards a research-based practice. Clinical governance is part of this move to achieve a critical mass.

As other chapters in this text highlight, clinical governance is a framework into which evidence-based practice, research, clinical effectiveness and clinical supervision (see Chapter 6) all fit. Proposed by policy makers to assure quality healthcare, this framework makes all healthcare professionals aware of their obligation to ensure that the care given is based on the best available evidence, that it is monitored and evaluated, that quality care is demonstrated and that a public account of practice is provided to patients, healthcare providers, purchasers and professionals.

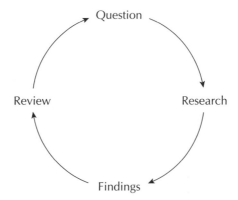

Figure 3.1 The cycle of evidence-based practice (adapted from Sackett *et al.,* 1996).

The development of clinical governance means that organizations must make a commitment to address the organizational, cultural and methodological barriers to evidence-based practice by investing in staff development and releasing practitioners for the purpose of research. A concentrated effort is required not only for the development of evidence-based practice but also for associated activities, for example clinical audit and quality assurance. The links between research, evidence-based practice and clinical governance, and in turn quality, are clear (see Fig. 3.1). The cycle of evidence-based practice could just as easily be the research cycle, specifically action research, and includes the key aspects of accountable practice and quality initiatives that clinical governance seeks to make explicit. So, how does evidence-based practice work in clinical practice? What follows is a more in-depth exploration of the stages of evidence-based practice, succeeded by a clinical case study demonstrating the application of theory to practice.

Giving care that is based on the best possible evidence

This entails accessing recent sources of literature, making use of existing standards and quality criteria developed from research or own experience, and searching for national clinical guidelines. It then follows that 'combination of results from clinically relevant research, clinical expertise and patient preferences produces the best evidence for insuring effective, individualized patient care' (Rosswurm and Larrabee, 1999: 317). However, any interpretation of evidence-based practice has to also take into account what is meant by clinical decision making (Walsh, 1998). The clinician is responsible for decision making and not all practice can be based purely on research (Sackett *et al.*, 1996). Where research and practice is not generalizable a consensus opinion should be sought.

Monitoring and evaluating care

This involves self-assessment through reflective practice, clinical supervision and the development of an ongoing professional dialog. Decisions need to be made as to who to include in the evaluation process, with particular attention to the role of partnerships and consumer involvement. This process of reflecting on practice enhances the development of explicit guidelines as opposed to measuring against implicit standards.

Demonstrating quality care

This involves seeking to maintain continuous quality improvement through audit and review in a multidisciplinary forum.

Public account of practice

At this stage practitioners are developing the skills of giving an account of practice. Professional practice is made open to scrutiny through the processes of reflective practice, clinical supervision, involvement of other disciplines and dissemination of research findings at local, national and international forums.

Case study

Outlined here is a brief clinical vignette which seeks to illuminate the stages of evidence-based practice adapted to a specific clinical setting.

The first skill that clinicians need to have before evidence-based practice or clinical effectiveness can even start to take place is the ability to question their own practice and to accept that there is possible room for improvement. Unless nurses automatically think each time they are about to be involved in clinical decision making – *Am I sure that I have the best available evidence to inform me and my patient when making this decision?* – evidence-based practice will only receive lip service. Obviously it is not possible for a practitioner to stop and carry out a literature search before each and every clinical decision is taken. However if, collectively, the clinical team consider where they are confident that evidence-based practice is taking place, then identify which areas they are less confident about and start to review these, eventually a culture of constant questioning will take place and evidence-based practice will be part and parcel of routine practice.

This is what has happened in one unit at a large acute NHS trust in the UK. The critical care unit at the acute hospital has set up a quality group in order to ensure that all practice is evidence based. The staff felt that practitioners were engaging in varying clinical practices, each approaching the caring situation differently and with no reference to a uniform standard. In addition, when new staff were appointed orientation was made difficult, as there were no explicit standards of practice on the unit. Increasingly staff were noticing a decline in their high standards of practice. As a result of this volunteers were asked to form the quality group with the remit of examining all clinical practices and working through those identified as priority, stage by stage. The group is multidisciplinary and consists of eleven members including specialist physicians and physical therapists. The group takes a full day out once a month to scrutinize relevant literature and to develop guidelines based on the best available evidence. The time-out day is funded from within the department itself and is counted within the members' working hours. Initially the group identified the clinical practices that were to be evidenced and are currently working on standards for invasive lines.

In order to pursue this, the group undertook a literature search and drew up guidelines for best evidence based on a systematic review (giving care that is based on the best possible evidence). So, questioning practice and defining the problem was the first step. When preparing for a literature search many librarians use the 'PICO' approach, that is, what is the Problem, what is the proposed Intervention, what is this being compared with (Comparison) and what is the intended Outcome? In the pursuit of evidence-based practice in nursing, nurses need to have an understanding of the different types of research and know how to appraise a published research article. They then need to be able to either take on board any suggested changes to their own practice or, where possible, influence the practice of others around them and finally be able to evaluate the impact of any such changes.

In the critical care unit, the guidelines, which then went out to peer review for comments to increase ownership, were put into practice and are currently being subjected to audit (three months later) (monitoring and evaluating care). An observational audit is being performed through the clinical effectiveness committee within the hospital to check that staff are adhering to the standard and a review date has been set (demonstrating quality care). It is envisaged that the standard will be reviewed annually in collaboration with the quality group. The results of clinical audit could be a possible source for evidence-based practice. This is particularly true in nursing where there are many gaps in the research evidence.

Every bed space in the unit has a copy of the guidelines, which are open to scrutiny by relatives and visitors; a copy is kept in the new staff orientation file; dissemination of the standards are trust-wide with copies being sent to the clinical effectiveness group and shared with the surgical directorate and recovery ward (public accountability of practice). As yet the standards have not been published or presented at national conferences because, as we were told, 'It's what everyone does, it's nothing special.'

The difference between evidence-based practice and clinical effectiveness is that whilst evidence-based practice involves identifying the problem, finding the evidence to inform what to do about the problem and then implementing these findings, clinical effectiveness means taking things a step further and evaluating the impact of implementation in order to inform future care. Making practice open to public scrutiny is part of moving evidence-based practice on to clinical effectiveness. This is achieved not only through writing for publication or presenting findings on relevant occasions, but also by ensuring that innovations in practice are closely monitored after implementation.

Having emphasized the increasing importance of research outcomes that are sensitive measures of nursing practice, it is vital that in the world of managed care, health care system variables as antecedents to outcomes demand increasing attention in nursing research.

To return to some of the questions posed at the beginning of this chapter, how can practitioners, educationalists, researchers, managers and policy makers work together to actualize these ideologies? We have already indicated that if nursing is to be evidence based it is necessary for a mechanism to be in place that allows and encourages the pursuit of this goal.

One of the most pressing problems in addressing this goal is that of narrowing the gap that prevails between theory, practice and more recently research in nursing. (For more detailed analysis of the theory–practice gap in relation to reflection, see Chapter 8.) It is true that changes are demanding that nurses, midwives and health visitors need to be able to seek out and apply evidence and as such it is essential that we improve the capability of the same to appraise and apply research findings to their practice (Bishop and Freshwater, 2004). Practitioners have to be empowered to identify outcomes that affect and influence care at the clinical level. However, systematic investigation of the practice of nursing is still a relatively new phenomenon in the nursing profession, even more so is the notion that the investigation is carried out by the practitioners themselves, that is 'practitioner-based research' (see Chapter 8 and Freshwater, 2004; Freshwater and Rolfe, 2001; Rolfe, 1998).

As much as nurses require training in research methods and data collection techniques, they also need to be re-educated to see that their nursing care can be translated into evidence and research findings. For as Rafferty and Traynor (1999) remind us, evidence does not travel one way only (researcher to practitioner): it is a two-way street. A number of contemporary initiatives have been developed that will tackle the issue of the practice–research gap and permit this two-way traffic, for example joint appointments, lecturer-practitioner and practitioner-researcher posts. Action research is also being more heavily utilized in order to bring occupational and organizational objectives closer together, thereby addressing the challenge of evidence-based practice. In deciding whether research findings are useful the practitioner has to evaluate whether their own personalized adaptation of the findings to a specific patient results in effective care. This means that all nurses are obliged to reflect on their practice and assess the effectiveness of the interventions that have been made and to consider whether the outcomes are satisfactory, both for the nurse and the patient. This in itself is research, for the research process is a method of posing questions about nursing practice and of seeking answers to them, as such research is a critical function for any profession that claims to base its practice on evidence. The move towards establishing nursing as an evidence-based profession will be achieved through evolution, not revolution, and demands long-term vision as well as short-term goals.

In this chapter it is proposed that the process of critically reflecting on evidence is a fundamental feature of empirical epistemology. It is further suggested that critical reflection on evidence derived from science, arts and humanities, and, in particular, practice experience can provide a sound basis for knowledge claims and the development of a science of practice for nursing and healthcare. It is argued that there is much to be gained by making the processes of critical reflection explicit, and that it can make a valid contribution to expert practice, without recourse to subjective or irreducible concepts such as intuition. The success of empirical science relies on a process of critically reflecting on evidence. The intent is to show that this process is similar to that used by practitioners to reflect on their practice through such media as supervision. Scientists and practitioners are being good empiricists by subjecting evidence from their experience to a critical thought process in a way that is open to scrutiny and contributes to a community of fellow thinkers. This process of critical reflection on the evidence is a familiar activity that draws upon a common and, to a large extent, recognizable logic of hypothetical reasoning (Freshwater and Avis, 2004; Gower, 1997). Hypothetical reasoning involves building or inventing hypotheses as plausible ways of explaining evidence from which we can deduce testable consequences. Simply stated, hypothetical reasoning starts from the question: *If this hypothesis could be justified then what consequences might be expected for our experiences and our theories?*

As evidence is generated through research or critical reflection, we use hypotheses as convenient explanatory beliefs to make sense of our experiences. These ideas may be tentative and somewhat vague at first, but as the process of reflection proceeds we attempt to give these beliefs more determinate content and specific connections with surrounding theory. We look to integrate these hypotheses into our web of beliefs, the scientific and cultural heritage of our community. An integral aspect of hypothesis testing includes prediction; we consider what kinds of evidence we might expect to obtain in the future if the hypothesis were true. These predictions help us decide whether a hypothesis is useful or not in explaining our experiences. Whether a working hypothesis should be accepted, revised or rejected is largely a pragmatic decision. Pragmatic criteria, such as consistency, convenience and simplicity, provide reasons to accept those hypotheses that help us to make the most sense of our experience in the context of our scientific and cultural heritage. In most cases a hypothesis will be accepted where it enhances consistency within our scientific and cultural system of beliefs, either by making new connections or confirming existing ones. However, this should not exclude the possibility that a hypothesis could be accepted that overturns existing conventions.

When hypothetical reasoning is applied to the process of critical reflection on evidence, we suggest that it is based on three identifiable steps. The process contains analytic procedures that use a hypothesis in order to reduce the evidence to its basic elements. In this sense a hypothesis is like a chemical reagent that causes other substances to appear – use of a hypothesis allows specific features of experience to become apparent. Critical reflection on the evidence also includes interpretation, using inductive logic to build new insights and conceptual explanations from the identification of basic elements of the evidence. Finally, we employ theory-testing procedures, deducing the consequences of new theoretical insights by examining their coherence with evidence (Freshwater and Avis, 2004). It must be stressed that the above steps are not intended to describe a straightforwardly sequential process; the process is iterative, idiosyncratic and cyclical.

Critical reflection as epistemology

One of the epistemological questions that remains is: can the hypotheses entertained during the process in critical reflection constitute knowledge? Holism about beliefs suggests that a hypothesis will become knowledge only if it can be established within a network of beliefs. It requires argument to demonstrate that accepting a particular hypothesis helps enlarge and improve our web of belief. Writers such as Rorty (1999) and Davidson (2001) argue that we should use pragmatic criteria such as convenience, simplicity, and resonance, in order to evaluate these arguments; arguments that provide good reasons to accept those hypotheses that help us to make the most sense of our experiences in the context of our particular scientific and cultural heritage. Arguments that enhance the consistency of our network of beliefs with the evidence from experience will lead us accept a hypothesis as true. Therefore, establishment of a hypothesis depends upon the quality of the argument that can be put forward to support the claim that it enhances the consistency of our network of beliefs.

The lingering shadow of positivism (as indicated in Chapter 2) can lead to the crude methodolatry that characterizes much quantitative research. This can be observed in claims about the hierarchy of methods and the validity of evidence; where empirical methods are based on slavish adherence to procedures designed to enhance reliability and validity of the data. Although these techniques seem to conventionally vouchsafe the quality of the evidence, they often fail to recognize the epistemological arguments needed to examine critically the nature of that evidence, especially when it is recognized that evidence cannot be isolated from a network of belief. It is the quality of the arguments that can be put forward to support a claim that matter most, although obviously the quality of the evidence will play some part in establishing that claim. In most cases a hypothesis will be accepted where it enhances consistency within our scientific and cultural system of beliefs, by making new connections, confirming existing ones, or by threatening to overturn them. Whether or not it is successfully established will still depend upon a pragmatic approach to weaving the hypothesis into a web of justification.

This does not imply that 'anything goes' for, as Rorty (1999) points out, no matter how much someone wishes to weave into their web of beliefs a private obsession or a matter of personal faith for which they cannot find adequate justification, the rest of their community will demand that they attend to any such contradiction. Rorty appears to accept that procedures of justification accepted within a community allow us to discard unhelpful concepts such as truth; however, it seems that if we find that a hypothesis is useful, consistent with our other beliefs, and improves the explanatory power of our network of belief then there is nothing much left to be anti-realist about.

Critical reflection as expert practice

It is fully acknowledged that judicious use of the results of good-quality research is a vital aspect of expert practice. The randomized controlled trial remains one of the best means we have to decide whether one form of care is better than another. However, a randomized controlled trial is simply an evaluation technique. Knowledge cannot be reduced to the application of a procedure. Knowing how to practice involves an understanding of the results of well-conducted research as well as an understanding of individuals and how to find out what they need; knowing how to practice involves sensitive application of contextual and idiosyncratic knowledge learnt through individual encounters with people.

Freshwater and Rolfe (2004) have observed that expert practice involves having to make decisions in a context where there is often incomplete evidence; and where there are no rules for the application of what evidence there is to an individual situation, and where the goal of intervention is resistant to scientific investigation, since it is value laden. In this circumstance we need to use *all* the evidence we have – from research, experience, the arts, and critical reflection to consider how to act. In short, we have to use the broader knowledge we possess. However, we also have to accept that knowledge is not immune from revision, and it derives from creative and critical thought on all the evidence we have amassed through reading and reflection. As a slogan, evidence-based practice is fine, but when it gets hijacked by positivists to argue that scientific evidence is the basis of practice we need to re-examine the usefulness of the concept.

It has been argued here that critical reflection on evidence is a fundamental aspect of expert practice, and that critical reflection on evidence has strong connections with the best traditions of empiricism.
The contention is that the process of critical reflection on evidence,
using the logic of hypothetical reasoning, finds strong connections
between the methods that qualitative and quantitative researchers as
well as expert practitioners use to justify the findings of their inquiries.
It should be observed that expert practice depends upon the use of
critical reflection to interpret a range of evidence in order to decide
how to act. This kind of complex and intricate evaluation of the evidence is quintessentially rational. Perhaps one of the reasons that
expert practice has been thought to be based on intuition is precisely
because the idea of rationality has been hijacked by the procedural,
methodical and instrumental reasoning regarded as synonymous with
a positivist epistemology.

If the question before practitioners is *what does the evidence indicate
about best practice in this context?* then reliable scientific evidence
must form part of the decision-making process, but it cannot decide
the matter on its own. The rational thought and debate with colleagues that is required to make a convincing case for action, using the
varieties of evidence at our disposal, cannot be reduced to following a
set of procedures. Equally, it should certainly not be placed in a black
box labeled 'intuition.' Best practice should be knowledge based, and
the most useful knowledge is that which is arrived at through a rigorous process of critical reflection on all the evidence we have obtained
through experience, reading novels, watching films, observing art and
reviewing scientific papers (Freshwater and Biley, 1998). What we
refer to here is what might be termed the 'burden of prudence,' in
which the researcher/practitioner/author is faced with their accountability, whether the emphasis is on the personal or professional. In
common to this position is the emphasis on the *person*hood of
the practitioner/researcher and the importance of self-reflection in the
production of reflective research texts.

Hence, a science of practice is one that draws heavily upon a pragmatic epistemology, which is grounded in practice, and based on the
premise that thought and action (in practice) are inseparable. This
view, which has been a central tenet of this chapter, is well rehearsed in
the nursing and education literature (e.g. Gibbs, 1988; Jarvis, 1996;
Rolfe, 1996; Usher and Bryant, 1989) and is neatly summarized by
Polkinghorne (2004: 5):

> *Practice is sometimes differentiated from theory, doing something
> as opposed to thinking about something. However, the distinction*

is overdrawn. Action and thought (both conscious and unconscious) are interactive. Practices are grounded in understandings people have about the world, and these understandings are, in turn, influenced by the effect of their practices on the world. Contemporary practice theory refocuses on the point of interaction of people with the world and others.

How a practitioner makes a decision about what to do in a particular clinical situation depends a lot on the individual: his/her assessment of the clinical situation/context, and his/her experience and exposure to different types of knowing. Thus, another important dimension of pragmatic epistemology is access to knowledge. For if practitioners are not exposed (or more importantly do not expose themselves) to new knowledge and do not access to their own knowledge through reflection, then they cannot use it for their practice.

Reflexive pragmatism is arguably an 'inclusive science of practice' in which practitioners are able to consider all forms of knowledge in terms of their suitability for application to their own practice; we suggest that advanced practitioners are more able to hold a 'creative tension' between formal and informal ways of knowing through such a prudent philosophy. It is an inverted philosophy, which cares for practice, rather than a caring philosophy.

References

Akinsanya, J. (1985) Learning about life. *Senior Nurse*, 2(5), 24–5.

Benner, P. (1984) *From Novice to Expert: Excellence and Power in Clinical Nursing Practice*. Addison-Wesley, Menlo Park, CA.

Bishop, V. and Freshwater, D. (2004) *Nursing Research in Context: Appreciation, Application and Professional Development*. Palgrave, Basingstoke, UK.

Brunning, H. and Huffington, C. (1985) Altered images. *Nursing Times*, 81(3), 24–7.

Capra, F. (1982) *The Turning Point, Society and the Rising Culture*. Fontana, London.

Chater, S. (1975) *Understanding Research in Nursing*. World Health Organization (WHO), Geneva.

Closs, J. and Cheater, F.M. (1996) Audit or research: what is the difference? *Journal of Clinical Nursing*, 5, 249–57.

Davidson, D. (2001) *Subjective, Intersubjective, Objective*. Oxford University Press, Oxford.

Fox, N.J. (1999) *Beyond Health, Postmodernism and Embodiment*. Free Association Books, London.

French, P. (1999) The development of evidence based nursing. *Journal of Advanced Nursing*, 29(1), 72–8.

Freshwater, D. and Avis, M. (2004) *Analyzing Interpretation and Reinterpreting Analysis*. Nursing Philosophy.

Freshwater, D. (2000) *Transformations learning in nurse education*. PhD Thesis, University of Nottingham, Nursing Praxis International.

Freshwater, D. and Biley, F. (1998) Rituals: the 'soul' purpose. *Complementary Therapies in Nursing and Midwifery*, 4(2), 73–6.

Freshwater, D. and Broughton, R. (2000) Research and evidence-based practice, in Bishop, V. and Scott, I. (eds) *Challenges in Clinical Practice: Professional Developments in Nursing*. Macmillan, London.

Freshwater, D. and Rolfe, G. (2001) Critical reflexivity: A politically and ethically engaged research method for nursing. *NT Research* (now *Journal of Nursing Research*), 6(1), 526–37.

Freshwater, D. and Rolfe, G. (2004) *Deconstructing Evidence Based Practice*. Routledge, London.

Friedson, E. (1970) *Professional Dominance*. Aldine Atherton, Chicago.

Gibbs, G. (1988) *Learning by Doing: A Guide to Teaching and Learning Methods*. Further Education Unit, Oxford Brookes University, Oxford.

Gower, B. (1997) *Scientific Method: An Historical and Philosophical Introduction*. Routledge, London.

Hicks, N. (1997) Evidence based healthcare. *Bandolier*, 4(39), 8.

Jarvis, P. (1996) The globalization of nurse education within higher education. *Nurse Education Today*, 17, 22–30.

Johns, C. and Hardy, H. (1998) Voice as a metaphor for transformation through reflection, in Johns, C. and Freshwater, D. (eds) *Transforming Nursing Through Reflective Practice*. Blackwell Science, Oxford.

Kelly, G.A. (1955) *The Psychology of Personal Constructs*. Norton, New York.

Kolb, D. (1984) *Experiential Learning*. Prentice-Hall, Englewood Cliffs, NJ.

Marks-Maran, D. (1999) Reconstructing nursing: evidence, artistry and the curriculum. *Nurse Education Today*, 19, 3–11.

Neville, B. (1989) *Educating Psyche*. Flat Chat Press, Greensborough, Australia.

Pfeiffer, J. and Jones, J. (1980) Structure experience Kit-users guide. California University Association. San Diego.

Poincaré, H. (1952) *Science and Method*. Dover Publications, New York.

Polkinghorne, D.E. (2004) *Practice and the Human Sciences: The Case for a Judgment-Based Practice of Care*. State University of New York Press, Albany, NY.

Rafferty, A.M. and Traynor, M. (1999) The research–practice gap in nursing: lessons from the research policy debate. *NT Research*, 4(6), 458–65.

Rolfe, G. (1996) *Closing the Theory–Practice Gap. A New Paradigm for Nursing*. Butterworth Heinemann, Oxford.

Rolfe, G. (1998) The theory–practice gap in nursing: from research-based practice to practitioner-based research. *Journal of Advanced Nursing*, 28(3), 672–9.

Rorty, R. (1999) *Philosophy and Social Hope*. Penguin, Harmondsworth, UK.

Rosenberg, W. and Donald, A. (1995) Evidence based medicine: an approach to clinical problem solving. *British Medical Journal*, 310(6987), 1122–6.

Rosswurm, M.A. and Larrabee, J.H. (1999) A model for change to evidence based practice. *Image: Journal of Nursing Scholarship*, 31(4), 317–22.

Sackett, D. and Rosenberg, W. (1995) On the need for evidence-based medicine. *Auditorium*, 2, 3–7.

Sackett, D.L., Rosenberg, W., Gray, J.A.M., Haynes, R.B. and Richardson, W.S. (1996) Evidence based medicine: what it is and what it isn't. *British Medical Journal*, 312, 71–2.

Salvage, J. (1998) Evidence based practice: a mixture of motives? *Nursing Times Research*, 3(6), 406–18.

Schön, D.A. (1983) *The Reflective Practitioner: How Practitioners Think in Action*. Basic Books, New York.

Usher, R. and Bryant, I. (1989) *Adult Education as Theory, Practice and Research: The Captive Triangle*. Routledge, London.

Wallas, G. (1926) *The Art of Thought*. Jonathan Cape, London.

Walsh, M.P. (1998) What is evidence? A critical view for nursing. *Clinical Effectiveness in Nursing*, 2, 86–93.

White, S.J. (1997) Evidence based practice and nursing: the new panacea? *British Journal of Nursing*, 6, 175–8.

Chapter 4

International perspectives in reflective practice: global knowledge reservoirs

Beverley J Taylor, Dawn Freshwater,
Gwen Sherwood and Philip Esterhuizen

Introduction

This chapter describes the history and applications of reflective practice across geographical and cultural boundaries, incorporating Australian, British, European, Asian and American perspectives, in an attempt to synthesize varying perspectives, contributing to the current status of reflective practice in nursing globally. Rather like Chapter 1, on the state of the art of reflection in nursing, it is certainly a bold promise to offer a global perspective on the status of reflective practice in nursing. This offer brings with it the difficulty of grasping the whole of a huge area and the danger of offending any people, who see themselves as being active influences in this area, who may be excluded or inadequately represented. Scholars' citations in literature, such as this chapter, now mean more than professional and academic recognition; they are also taken to indicate research quality and impact, with real dollar values attached to academic institutions. Therefore, at the outset of undertaking this immense task, it is important to clarify our assumptions about nursing literature, history and cultures, as we attempt to offer in this chapter international perspectives of reflective practice in nursing.

Reflection in the nursing literature

Nursing literature relating directly to reflective practice has experienced a sustained growth globally since the mid 1980s, beginning its influence in Australia, moving through literature sources and professional conference discourses to the UK and other parts of the world. The literature has been disseminated mainly through refereed journal articles in hard copy and, more recently, in full-text online articles, which provide the quickest turn-around time in the publication process, allowing for more immediate readers' responses. Books have also been important literature sources, especially in nurse education, research and management, as guides for nursing practice within complex healthcare systems. Professional conference proceedings have also been influential literature sources in sharing ideas on reflective practice in nursing.

Nursing in Australia, UK, Europe and Asia has witnessed a boom in scholarship in the last two to three decades, as a direct result of the movement of nurse education into tertiary settings, such as colleges of advanced education and universities. Until the 1980s, these countries relied on nursing scholarship and postgraduate nurse education generated mainly in the USA and Canada, where various systems of nurse education have been demonstrating high standards of research-based disciplinary status since the 1920s. Many Australian, British, European and Asian nurses undertaking post-registration study at various levels have at some time studied the work of the North American nurse theorists, and have been required to apply these ideas to nursing practice, education, research and management.

With the advent of tertiary nurse education came the academic imperatives to undertake research, publish research and scholarly articles, teach from research-based evidence, and develop disciplinary status through professional and community development activities. These academic catalysts created national contributions to nursing scholarship in local refereed journals, books and monograph series, and professional discourses were also established through presentations and debates at national and international nursing conferences. Therefore, although Australian, British, European and Asian nurses still respected and studied North American scholarship, they began to amass in their own professional literature pertaining to their perspectives of nursing practice, research, education and management. Global changes, such as international travel and technological advances, including the World Wide Web, email and videoconferencing, have made the world of nursing smaller and easier to traverse, literature is increasingly non-paper-based and nurse scholars are moving beyond ethnocentric views to encompass global perspectives of nursing.

In this chapter, we assume that the history of reflective practice in nursing is embodied in its participants, who provide their oral histories of living through changes in nurse education in the last 20 years or so. No formal research project has been undertaken to write this chapter, as it would have been an undertaking of postgraduate research proportions, to do justice to tracking and capturing descriptions of reflective practice in nursing worldwide. History varies according to the person telling the account, so we assume that the authors' views of history may vary from other people's perspectives. Therefore, with as much comprehensiveness as possible, this chapter assumes that the history of reflective practice in nursing can only be a relative and partial account, told through the perspectives of the authors of this chapter, with reference to some of the literature emanating from various countries.

This leads to our assumptions about cultures, which we assume to be 'embedded' cultures, in the sense that we can only imagine and attempt to represent the symbols, rituals and nursing practices of groups of people who, for the time, find themselves embedded within defined national borders. Geographical boundaries have less meaning in nursing scholarship than ever before, as researchers and scholars live in other countries for months to years at a time, collaborate on international projects, become active members of international professional organizations, and present their work at international conferences in person and online. Therefore, nursing cultures take on non-fixed, integrated perspectives that do not necessarily denote geographical boundaries or national identities. The internationalization of nursing scholarship and the multicultural nature of countries around the globe defy the articulation of national identities that do not resort to stereotypical cultural descriptions. With these assumptions about literature, history and culture in mind, and apologies to anyone who may feel excluded or under-represented, we attempt to describe the history of reflective practice in nursing from our perspectives.

Australian and New Zealand perspectives

Although Australia and New Zealand are two very different countries, with their own national histories, politics and systems of nursing and nurse education, they nevertheless share many initiatives in nursing scholarship. Australia and New Zealand have been combined in this section, due to mixing of nursing perspectives, enhanced by frequent international air travel across the relatively short distance of the Tasman Sea, referred to jokingly in both countries as 'the Ditch'; respect for one another through the ANZAC wartime tradition; the collaborative activities of international nursing committees, such as the Australian and New Zealand Deans of Nursing; and the fact that many Australian nurses live and work in New Zealand and vice versa.

A telling of the history

Bev Taylor identifies as Australian, so she will relate the history and trends of reflective practice from her perspective of living the last 20 years or so in Australia, realizing that other nurses in Australia and New Zealand may see it differently. Scholarship in reflective practice began in the southern hemisphere within the discipline of education at Deakin University, Australia, informed mainly by the work of Donald Schön (1983) and Jurgen Habermas (1973). Established as a university in 1977, Deakin University attracted many important educationalists, who pioneered reflective practice for teachers. Among these luminaries were Stephen Kemmis, John Smyth, Robin McTaggart and Annette Street. In the late 1970s to early 1980s, many nurses undertaking postgraduate degrees needed to take their studies outside nursing in established non-nursing disciplines. Hospital-based certificate programs in nursing did not cease intakes of student nurses until 1985, when most States and Territories began the transfer of nurse education to colleges of advanced education. Therefore, nurses often graduated with postgraduate degrees from other disciplines, such as a Master of Education.

In 1987, Professor Alan Pearson was appointed as Foundation Chair at the Faculty of Nursing, Deakin University, Geelong. He set up the faculty with a focus on the centrality of practice, recruiting staff with clinical expertise and/or with a strong commitment to nursing practice. The first year witnessed rapid faculty growth, which involved setting up clinical networks and programs and initiating research-informed practice-based teaching from undergraduate to doctoral levels, and the establishment of a research centre and professorial nursing practice units. Staff development included workshops in reflective practice, facilitated by Dr Annette Street, who, as an educator in the Faculty of Education at Deakin University, had already guided some Faculty of Nursing staff in reflective practice studies through distance education programs. Other influential scholars in education at that time, who shared their knowledge and skills with nurses, were Stephen Kemmis and John Smyth. The interest in reflective practice in Australian nursing sprang directly from these three people in particular and the positive influence they had through the study of education at Deakin University at that time. Thus, reflective practice applied itself readily to nurse education and practice in Australia, facilitated by the Faculty of Nursing at Deakin University from 1987. Now, reflective practice is fundamental to Australian clinical nursing practice and education and it is also used in research projects. Given the relatively long life of Australian reflective practice in nursing, the current challenge relates to maintaining enthusiasm and depth of engagement in reflective processes.

Examples of scholarship

Applying the ideas of 'knowing-in-action' offered to teachers by Kemmis (1985) and praxis as change through reflection (Nias, 1987; Smyth, 1987; Tripp, 1987), Australian and New Zealand nurses began to consider their 'theories-of-action' to reflect on the differences between what they espoused and what they actually did in their work. Influential writing of that time, often expressed in the language of critical social science, included Perry's (1985) 'reflexive critique of conceptions and experiences of theory and practice in the induction of five graduate nurses' (Moss, 2004: 36), Street's PhD thesis (1989), 'Thinking, Acting and Reflecting,' and her subsequent works published as monographs (Street, 1990, 1991, 1992). Street's latest publications use reflection as central to research processes in critical ethnography (e.g. Wellard and Street, 1999). Other early writers in critical social science as it applied to praxis in nursing were Cox (Cox, 1990; Cox and Moss, 1988; Cox *et al.*, 1991), Hickson (1988, 1990), Clare (formerly Perry) (1991), Moss (Cox and Moss, 1988; Perry and Moss, 1988), Emden (1991), Lumby (1991) and Dixon (1996). These earliest Australian and New Zealand publications offered a critical social science perspective, encouraging nurses to reflect systematically on the status quo within nursing to identify the reified constraints and other causes of false consciousness, to take collaborative action to transform the oppressive structures of the healthcare system. This theme was written into literature and applied in nursing curricula throughout Australia and New Zealand as an overtly political agenda, although the extent to which this has been effective in causing change has been questioned since those heady days of 'revolution' in the form of transformative practice in nursing (Clinton, 1998; Taylor, 1997; Usher and Holmes, 2006).

The Gray and Pratt (1989, 1991, 1992, 1995) series of books played a significant role in the emerging identity of Australian and New Zealand nurse scholarship. One of the most influential publications on reflective practice was written by three colleagues working at Deakin University (Cox *et al.*, 1991). In this book chapter Cox *et al.* (1991) explore reflection as knowing and constructing practice and come to the conclusion that:

> *the knowledge nurses generate in and through their practice con-tributes to the discipline of nursing, because practice lies at the heart of nursing and it is by illuminating and articulating this dynamic core that the nature of nursing can be made explicit.* (Cox *et al.*, in Gray and Pratt, 1991: 388)

Greenwood (1998) identified the role of reflection in single loop and double loop learning (we referred to Greenwood's work in Chapter 1). In single loop learning, the level of response is to simply change the actions intended to lead to the same outcomes. In double loop learning the person uses values and norms to examine the appropriateness and correctness of the chosen end. Smyth's (1992) framework is explicitly double loop. Greenwood asserts that the former frameworks may be most suited for young learners with limited experience, whereas the latter is recommended for reflective practice that incorporates the norms, values and social relationships which underpin human action.

More recent Australian and New Zealand examples of reflective prac-tice research and scholarship include Taylor's book (2006) describing and applying three main types of reflection – technical, practical and emancipatory – based on Habermas's (1973) knowledge constitutive interests. The types of reflection are categorized according to the kind of knowledge they involve and the work interests they represent. Technical reflection based on the scientific method and rational, deductive thinking allows nurses to generate and validate empirical knowledge through rigorous means, so that they can be assured that work procedures are based on scientific reasoning. Practical reflection leads to interpretation for description and explanation of human interactions in social settings. Emancipatory reflection leads to 'trans-formative action,' which seeks to free nurses from taken-for-granted assumptions and oppressive forces, which limit them and their prac-tice. Other contributions to reflective practice scholarship include research using action research and reflection (Taylor, 2001; Taylor *et al.*, 2002, 2005) and refereed articles about the application of reflective practice in nursing and holistic healthcare settings (Taylor, 2002, 2003, 2004).

Other contributions to scholarship in reflective practice in Australia and New Zealand include Teekman (2000), Peerson and Yong (2003) and Levett-Jones (2007). Teekman (2000) used the qualitative research method of sense-making, to explore with ten Registered Nurses their reflective thinking in actual nursing practice. He observed that

> *Reflective thinking was extensively manifest, especially in moments of doubt and perplexity, and consisted of such cognitive activities as comparing and contrasting phenomena, recognizing patterns, categorizing perceptions, framing, and self-questioning in order to create meaning and understanding.* (Teekman, 2000: 1125)

Peerson and Yong (2003) explored reflexivity in nursing and questioned the location of the patient and the nurse. The article probed four issues relative to nursing practice: 'seeking technological solutions to health and ill-health; moving from the nurse–patient relationship to the patient–healer relationship; utilizing critical pathways; and supporting evidence-based nursing' (Peerson and Yong, 2003: 30). The authors agreed that we

> *need to encourage nurses to engage in reflexivity and not to lose sight of their selves (knowledge, expertise and skills), and their patients' voices and subjectivity in their contribution to health care.* (Peerson and Yong, 2003: 30)

Levett-Jones (2007) described the use of narratives to self-assess nursing competence. She concluded that narrative reflection

> *allows students to go well beyond a detailed description of an episode of their practice, to an in-depth analysis of, and reflection on, the meaning of the episode. The power of narrative reflection is its potential to enhance student's ability to critique and learn from practice, develop clinical competence, and articulate, appreciate and value their practice.* (Levett-Jones, 2007: 118)

Critiques of reflective practice emerged over time. For example, Greenwood (1993) provided a critique of Schön's model of reflection-on-action and reflection-in-action, claiming that it failed to recognize the importance of reflection-before-action. Reflection before action involves thinking through what one wants to do and how one intends to do it before one actually does it. This relates closely to mindfulness where one discharges judgments or biases and opens oneself to the moment, by clearing out unwanted distractions and eliciting presence and openness before interacting with others.

Other notes of caution were sounded, for example, Taylor (1997) warned nurse teachers of the problems associated with 'big battles for small gains,' because emancipatory reflective processes encourage nurses to question taken-for-granted assumptions and structures, and in attempting to be transformative, nurses may incur the wrath of powerful people within systems of healthcare.

Clinton (1998) questioned the possibility of nurses actually achieving reflection-in-action with the argument:

> *(i) that nurses cannot be conscious of all aspects of nursing practice because there are aspects of practice that cannot be represented in consciousness, (ii) that those aspects of practice that can be represented in consciousness can be so only imperfectly, (iii) that all such representations are not reflexive, and (iv) that any representation in the form of an internal dialogue that could be regarded as reflection is overdetermined.* (Clinton, 1998: 197)

Usher and Holmes (2006) provided a comprehensive overview of reflective practice, including the critiques, that it remains ill-defined, that it is a surveillance method for private thoughts, that it masquerades as radical, even though it imposes a 'standardised way of thinking and acting,' and 'not enough attention has been paid to the negative aspects of reflection' and of 'trying to be a reflective practitioner' (Usher and Holmes, 2006: 112). Even so, they provide a counterbalance to the criticisms by suggesting

- the meaning of words is a matter of convention, and agreement takes time to emerge;
- self-scrutiny is a positive feature of professional life; indeed 'profession' is often characterized by such self-regulation;
- the aim is to open up practitioners' minds to possibilities, not to impose rules, and reflective practitioners are therefore more likely to be creative, to challenge the status quo, and to be independent thinkers; and
- the problems of reflective practice may have been underestimated, but they are increasingly acknowledged; in any case, this means that we need to be better at reflective processes, not that they should be abandoned (Usher and Holmes, 2006: 112).

In summary, the Australian and New Zealand perspective of reflective practice in nursing began in the mid 1980s at Deakin University, influenced and supported strongly by Stephen Kemmis, John Smyth, Robin McTaggart and Annette Street. Professor Alan Pearson, as Foundation Chair of the Faculty of Nursing, Deakin University, Geelong, established many practice-based initiatives, including reflective practice for staff and students. From this beginning point, reflective practice has become enshrined in many nursing curricula throughout Australia and New Zealand and the scholarship has been mainly in the areas of nurse education and nursing practice and research.

British perspectives

A telling of the history

Nursing in the United Kingdom, along with other professions, has seen a dramatic interest and increase in the potential of reflection as a learning tool and as a means of integrating theory and practice (Atkins and Murphy, 1993; Clarke, 1986; Osbourne, 1996; Schön, 1983). Historically, the UK has done much to progress and expand the literature and research in this area, although much of the early work around reflection was deliberative and there still continues debate over what constitutes reflective practice per se (Atkins and Murphy, 1993; Boyd and Fales, 1983; Palmer *et al.*, 1994; Ghaye and Ghaye, 1998; Johns and Freshwater, 1998, 2005; Rolfe *et al.*, 2001; and many others). Building on the work of educationalist Donald Schön and philosopher James Dewey, numerous UK practitioners have, over the last 30 years, created a fairly robust and substantial evidence base.

Chris Johns was one of the early influential thinkers in the area of reflective practice, developing a model of best practice in the Burford Nursing Development Unit. Johns (1995) interprets reflection as being:

> *the practitioner's ability to access, makes sense of and learn through work experience, to achieve more desirable, effective and satisfying work.* (p. 24)

Johns set up and has spearheaded the internationally known annual reflective practice conference, which has had a significant impact on the scholarship, dissemination and practice of reflection. Indeed the text *Transforming Nursing through Reflective Practice* originated from this conference in 1998 and has done much to inform and support the growing community of advocates of reflection. Johns' models of reflection have evolved considerably since his first iteration, and continue to be used widely nationally and internationally. At the same time Anthony Bulman, Della Fish, Gary Rolfe, Melanie Jasper, Dawn Freshwater and Tony Ghaye were all also focussing energies on aspects of reflection and its application to nursing research, nurse education, nursing practice and leadership. Rolfe and Jasper in particular have significantly impacted the way in which reflection is viewed as a tool for advanced practice and portfolio development. Both Johns and Freshwater have integrated reflection with caring theories, with Freshwater emphasizing the role of reflection in supervisory and research processes. She has attended in the main to the therapeutic use of self and the intersubjective nature of reflective processes. Along with Rolfe, she continues to scrutinize the nature of reflexivity, interrogating it in parallel with the concept of evidence-based practice (Freshwater and Rolfe, 2001, 2004; Rolfe, 1998).

For Johns the issue of concern that is fundamental to the process of reflection from the experience of conflict in practice. This was also the thrust of the work of Argyris and Schön (1974) who discussed the notion of action theories. All human actions reflect ideas, models or some kind of theoretical notion of purpose and intention and how these purposes and intentions can be executed (Freshwater, 1998; Langford, 1973). These notions can be called action theories. Argyris and Schön (1974) noted that people often say one thing and do another. Thus, an individual has a personal theory but when it is operationalized, there is often a contradiction. Based on this idea, Argyris and Schön (1974) developed the concept of espoused theories, the stated purpose or intention, and theories in use, the attempt to put stated intentions or purpose into action. Espoused theories are those to which individuals claim allegiance: theories in use are those theories which are present when action is executed. Human action therefore is never atheoretical or accidental, even if the theory involved in the action is implicit or tacit. It is argued that reflection is a way of redeeming theories in use which may be tacit. (There is clearly an overlap here with the Australian literature; see for example Greenwood, 1998.)

Most of the UK literature on reflection and critical reflection takes a longitudinal view, one that is based within a linear timeframe, drawing upon Western logic. Although more recently authors are relating the reflective process to Eastern traditions such as Buddhism (Johns), mindfulness and meditation (Freshwater).

Examples of scholarship

There is some evidence, albeit minimal, that reflective practice has links with client outcomes. Powell (1989) attempted to access tacit knowledge, often described as defying explanation, using reflection. Powell's (1989) study used Mezirow's levels of reflectivity as signposts to monitor the depth of reflection undertaken by a group of practitioners. Although a small sample was used in this local study, it provides a useful benchmark for development to explore how levels of reflection may enhance practice outcomes. Other research studies that have examined the link between reflection and client care include McCaugherty (1991), Johns (1998), Houston (1995) and Freshwater (1998).

Much of the research that has explored reflective practice as a teaching and learning tool in nursing has been carried out with post registration nurses (Powell, 1989; Richardson and Maltby, 1995). Rationale for this is often around the point made earlier concerning the ability of student nurses to make use of reflection as a learning process. David McCaugherty (1991), however, examined a teaching model to promote reflection with first year student nurses in the clinical area. Freshwater (1998) conducted a longitudinal study of developing a reflective curriculum. Over the past two decades, the implementation of clinical supervision has shifted the focus of the scholarship of reflective practice; much of this is reported in Chapter 6 and is extensive.

Atkins and Murphy (1993), for example, undertook a review of the literature on reflection and concluded that the available literature is complex and abstract. It is the legacy of the traditional positivist paradigm that drives us to know exactly what reflection is, knowing the thing that we work with enables us to control and manipulate it to certain ends. Nevertheless there has been a considerable amount of UK literature produced on the subject and it is an important part of the process to explore the development of our knowledge of reflection thus far.

European perspectives

A Dutch perspective

A telling of the history

In general, reflection in the Netherlands developed from a learning psychology perspective – more specifically from a humanistic paradigm. In essence those supporting this approach suggested that an individual learns out of free will and has a desire for self-actualization and self-realization, which includes creativity. The most essential factor is their motivation for inner growth which is considered to be a fundamental desire – even if there are environmental factors which could block this development (Hilgard and Atkinson, 1979). Also influential was the notion of constructivism and the way an activity develops; in other words, understanding which actions underpin the way in which a student reaches an answer (Span, 1987; Van Parreren, 1987). The idea behind this approach is that the outcomes are fixed, but that it is the process the student follows to reach the outcomes that is of significance. Work by Vermunt (1992) was important in developing awareness of reflection as a method of learning, defining learning as a metacognitive skill through which an individual develops new knowledge and insight due to their analyzing an experience (OLVG, 2001).

The developments that took place resulted in a structural and prescriptive approach to reflection within the Dutch context. Work by Koetsenruiter *et al.* (2001) is described as a handbook for reflection and includes numerous instruments and models for use by nurses. Hesselink (2004) and Benammar (2004: 2) provided workshops and training sessions for educators, suggesting

> *it is our intention to provoke reflection from students, to give structure to this process and, also to assess whether reflection has occurred or not.*

However, not all work in the Netherlands at this time was prescriptive. Mensink (1996) and Venneman and Arends (2001) challenged educators and clinicians to reflect on practice and highlighted the enrichment associated with reflective practice. And in challenging the positivist status quo, Strijbol (1996) used reflective narrative to critique nursing responsibility and care. Simultaneously reflective challenges were being introduced into books listed in compulsory reading lists for different levels of nursing program (Achterberg *et al.*, 2002; Esterhuizen, 2002; Van de Wiel and Woude, 2000).

Looking back over the past two decades one realizes that, in broad terms, reflection, reflective practice and reflexivity as described in international literature are still in their infancy in the Netherlands. Although there have been pockets of development in the area of reflection and reflective practice, development has been slightly different to the process in English-speaking countries and, to date, these have not been harnessed or used collectively to develop a cohesive body of knowledge. This could be due to the individuality and rationality of the Dutch culture, but it could also be related to the strength of the dominant, positivist discourse still prescriptive towards clinical, education and research activities.

North American perspectives

A telling of the history

The scholarship of reflective practice continues to be in an emergent state in North American nursing. Historically, applications of reflection based on models from the United Kingdom were primarily cited as an abstract teaching strategy for students to give thoughtful consideration of a particular experience. In general, reflection has often lacked the established systems and processes as explicated in Australia, New Zealand and the UK with little application towards clinical supervision and research applications. Related systematic thinking processes, however, are integral to effective nursing practice, education, research and management and have an increasing role in North American nursing scholarship. Applications will be examined within knowledge development, practice, education and organizational impacts as well as a section on scholarship development.

The influence of reflection on the development of American nursing is often more implicit than explicit. American caring theories illustrate the implicit influence of a reflective stance in the advancement of nursing knowledge. The development of nursing theories and models helped to organize nursing knowledge in orderly, coherent ways to provide descriptions and maps for thoughtful practice, blending theory and practice perspectives. Theorists such as Peplau (1952), Paterson and Zderad (1976), Leininger (1978), Watson (1979), Benner (1984), Newman (1986) and Boykin and Schoenhofer (2001) grounded their work in a human becoming perspective that requires a thoughtful, reflective practice orientation. Practice models derived from these theories engage the nurse in knowing the self as a therapeutic agent, bringing the reflective self into practice. These familiar works are among those described briefly in Chapter 11 and demonstrate the profound contributions American nurse scholars have made to the organization of nursing knowledge worldwide.

Benner's (1984) work is pre-eminent in developing nursing practice by using practitioner descriptions of expertise and the knowledge embedded in expert nursing practice. Using paradigm cases around patient care issues, Benner (1984) defined nursing practice as movement from novice to expert and concluded that 'a wealth of untapped knowledge is embedded in the practices and the "know-how" of expert nurse clinicians' and that nurses need to 'systematically record what they learn from their own experience.' The systems and processes of established reflective practice provide the means of recording and making sense of clinical experiences, thus ensuring that 'know-how' contributes to disciplinary knowledge. Benner (1984) uses reflective narratives, called exemplars, to help practitioners understand the implications of the illness experience from the patient perspective, bringing higher levels of expertise to the care experience by bridging theory and practice. Benner (1984) uses 'thinking-in-action' to make reflective processes more explicit, to help practitioners engage in their practice. Moss (2004) aligns this approach with Schön's (1983) ideas about 'knowing-in-action' and 'reflection-in-action' and the 'theories-of-action' literature.

The impact of reflection is most evident in American nursing educa-tion through critical thinking. It may be that reflection as an edu-cational influence grew as a reaction to the 'technical rationality and competence-based initiatives' that dominated nursing in the 1970s and 1980s (Ruth-Sahd, 2003). Bevis (1989) called for a curriculum revolution to move away from the prescriptive models guided by beha-vioral objectives that defined the dominant content-driven approach. Bevis called for open space models that were learner-centered in which students observed a practice area, reflected on what knowledge would be needed to care for a particular population of patients, and used self-guided learning models in which students shared what they learned. Faculty were facilitators rather than deliverers of know-ledge. The goal was to change behavior by creating a spirit of inquiry in students so that their practice becomes a constant seeking of evi-dence of the best way to accomplish care goals (Bevis and Watson, 1989). Cranton (1996) placed reflection as the cornerstone of trans-formative learning, the action step towards a change in behavior.

While Bevis's open space learning had limited lasting influence on how nursing is taught, evaluated and credentialed, current redesign in nursing education is applying curricula models and pedagogies which embrace reflection and capture the spirit of Bevis's model. Most evident are curricula based on the caring theories mentioned above. These curricula are characterized by reflective student learning experi-ences built around Carper's (1978) four ways of knowing: empirical, personal, ethical, and aesthetic. Boykin and Schoenhofer (2001) describe a caring-based curriculum with a goal of 'an ongoing creation of nursing through experience.' Two core ingredients include the ways of knowing and alternating rhythms which is defined as moving back and forth between action and reflection. Chinn and Watson (1994) apply aesthetics as a basis for developing moral, ethical and personal ways of knowing. Reflection is woven throughout a widely adopted textbook on holistic nursing (Dossey *et al.*, 2000). Self-reflection allows the connection of mind, body and spirit for a holistic caring process. Learning strategies include diaries, journals, intuition logs, mind maps, story, music and life review.

A sampling of recent nursing literatures demonstrates that reflection is most often applied in American nursing as a teaching learning strategy (Ruth-Sahd, 2003). Reflective writing and journaling are used to develop critical thinking (Croke, 2004; Forneris and Peden-McAlpine, 2007; Kennison, 2006; Kessler and Lund, 2004), transform the professional practice perspectives of RN-BSN students (Ruland and Ahern, 2007), and monitor student progress towards personal knowing and critical thinking in online nursing courses (Hermann, 2006; Kessler and Lund, 2004). Jensen and Joy (2005) and Kennison (2006) developed methods for evaluating reflection in student journals. Parker (1994) used guided reflection as students work with clay as a centering, mindful reflection-on-action. Sherwood (1997) developed a guided reflection for students to complete after viewing a mainstream movie to apply lessons for spiritual development. Reflection is the basis for using story (Branch and Anderson, 1999) that can be applied in work with patients as well as for providers in understanding self within the experience. Drevdahl *et al.* (2002) merged reflective inquiry and self-study to enable teachers to better understand themselves as teachers as well as how their teaching affects students.

Reflection is cited as a major instructional strategy in new paradigms around quality and safety, now the focus in American healthcare. In the wake of staggering reports of poor healthcare outcomes from the Institute of Medicine (IoM), healthcare professions education is under redesign to address quality and safety content (IoM, 2001). Goals for cross-disciplinary education are based on five competencies that include patient-centered care, teamwork and collaboration, evidence-based practice, quality and safety, and informatics. To achieve these competencies, the IoM study group called for reflective pedagogies across the professions to achieve behavior change. Across the disciplines, healthcare practitioners must be able to systematically integrate didactic learning with experiential learning from a reflective process for a more contemplative understanding of the patients' illness experience (IoM, 2003).

A national project by Cronenwett *et al.* (2007) further defined these competencies with knowledge, skills and attitudes for transforming nursing education. Integration of these competencies into professional identity formation will contribute to a quality and safety culture as the framework for practice. Working from a spirit of inquiry requires a reflective stance that constantly questions how theory and experience are linked, how care can be improved, what is the source of the next possible adverse event, and what are areas needing quality improvement initiatives within the work group (Sherwood and Drenkard, 2007). Honoring this kind of reflective practice stems from a system perspective that moves from 'the way we always have done it' to systematically and reflectively thinking about what we do, how we do it, and how we can improve the system to change patient care outcomes.

There is a resurgent interest in the pedagogies previously proposed by Bevis (1989; Bevis and Watson, 1989) which build on reflection. The knowledge, skills and attitudes of the quality and safety competencies require reflective teaching pedagogies (Day and Smith, 2007; Sherwood and Drenkard, 2007) to fill the gap between traditional education and expectations in healthcare systems with a quality and safety culture. Emotional intelligence is the cornerstone for these competencies (Cronenwett *et al.*, 2007). Applications of reflection for expanding leadership capacity in American nursing are detailed in Chapter 7. Most notably is application of reflection for emotional intelligence as healthcare professionals develop self-discovery, self-awareness, self-management, motivation to contribute to something larger than oneself, and empathy for others' situation (Cherniss and Goleman, 2001; Vitello-Cicciu, 2002).

The role of reflection in effective change agency is another area of emergence in American nursing. Increasing attention to the environment in which nurses work (IOM, 2003) has led to analysis of contextual and situational factors which impact on how nurses respond. Managers and organizational leaders seek methods for building a work culture that appreciates and values the expertise and input from nurses (Havens *et al.*, 2006). Appreciative Inquiry (AI) is a philosophy as well as an analysis and change process which focusses on successes, values and dreams rather than gap analysis (Keefe and Pesut, 2004). AI, like reflection, derives from asking questions about experiences. Asking questions begins the change process. Appreciative Inquiry helps clarify assumptions and beliefs so that goals for change are allowed to emerge. Appreciative Inquiry is built on the principle of appreciating or valuing to affirm strengths, successes and stories that give life to a system. Inquiry uses questions to seek new potentials and possibilities by engaging participants in reflective discovery to co-create their desired work environment.

Using a reflective framework, the four cycles of AI include (Keefe and Pesut, 2004):

1 Discovery: reflecting and sharing stories that illustrate values, things appreciated, and what makes a system work.
2 Dream: reflective questions challenge the status quo by looking at what we have and could be to envision something new.
3 Design: reflects on how something can be by co-constructing a course of action to gain a preferred future.
4 Delivery: reflecting and sharing what each will do to help realize the dream envisioned and how feedback loops will ensure lasting change.

Examples of scholarship

Advancement of nursing science in the United States emphasized empirical knowledge development with little attention to the inner reflections that uncover meaning in experience, the personal, ethical, and aesthetic ways of knowing (Carper, 1978). With Watson's call for a paradigm shift through 'a new scientific quest' (1981), other research methodologies began to emerge. While early in nursing science development, qualitative approaches such as phenomenology, naturalistic inquiry, and grounded theory were largely ignored and thought to be 'soft science,' they have slowly gained acceptance within the mainstream of North American nursing research as a way of collecting evidence, understanding experience, and developing theory.

Reflection is consistent with the goals of qualitative research and many nursing studies utilize a reflective framework to guide participants into closer examination of their healthcare experiences. A series of progressively deeper questions that reflect-on-action can also guide healthcare professionals in analysis of a case study to uncover role delineation, responses to difficult cases, and thinking about patient provider interactions (Sherwood, 2000). Narrative techniques are useful for encouraging patients to make sense of their illness episode as a caring–healing strategy (Sakalys, 2003). Cohen *et al.* (2000) used story to guide patient reflections on the deeper meaning of bone marrow transplant, an example of helping patients reflect-in-action, that is within the experience as it is unfolding to find meaning and purpose.

Reflective models can guide theory development. Using phenomenology, Swanson (1991) interviewed patients who miscarried to develop a middle range theory of caring. In Horton-Deutsch and Horton's (2003) grounded theory study mindfulness is cited as the basic social process that leads to working through difficult communicative situations. Mindfulness, or awareness and insight, is a state of being purposefully attentive to one's moment-to-moment experience (O-Haver

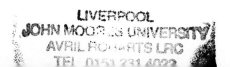

Day and Horton-Deutsch, 2004). This idea aligns with 'reflection-in-action,' as it involves paying attention, on purpose, to one's own thoughts, feelings, bodily sensations and judgments. Much like the reflective transformative processes detailed in Chapter 7, mindfulness helps nurses to be more aware of communication within themselves and with others, develop insight into how perceptions shape actions, identify and understand other people's standpoints, and to respond effectively.

Mindfulness requires individuals to take the stance of a detached observer, to become fully aware of perceptual experiences, and create a sense of balance and tolerance for one's conscious experience (O-Haver Day and Horton-Deutsch, 2004). A similar application uses mindfulness as the intervention in therapeutic communities (Marcus *et al.*, 2007). The detached stance enables mindful responses, rather than habitual behaviors that might perpetuate and intensify situations, much like the reflection required in developing emotional intelligence (Vitello-Cicciu, 2002). Mindfulness applies the skills in counseling, meditation, breathing and relaxation to respond calmly and purposively to potentially inflammatory communicative situations, with compassion, empathy and openness.

Reflection as applied in the US, then, is in an emergent state as illustrated in the growth of applications in practice, curriculum, pedagogy, change management and scholarship. Interventions based on reflective processes such as mindfulness continue to be developed and measured. Still, we in the US continue to learn from our global colleagues new applications of reflection applications for clinical supervision. While there is increasing use of professional practice models and portfolios for evaluation of individual practitioners, reflection remains in abstract and limited application in practice settings. Evaluation and outcome measures of its effectiveness remains an elusive challenge to determine most effective ways to prepare for new paradigms of care, education, and research in the US. Sound effective assessments could impact the continuing immersion of reflection in advancing all areas of nursing scholarship.

Summary

Reflective practice has become part of the discourse of nursing education classrooms, continuing education, research design and teacher preparation. Reflective practice still remains disparate, with many forms and applications throughout the world. The varying approaches and applications of reflection in multiple geographic regions illustrate common themes as well as differences. Here we attempt to synthesize the varying perspectives and contributions of reflection to show the widespread use and how no one paradigm dominates. In nursing we continue to advance our understanding of the definition, application, integration and evaluation of reflective methods. Clearly the leadership from Australia, New Zealand, and the United Kingdom has influenced the emergence of reflection in North America and Europe.

References

Achterberg, T., Eliens, A. and Strijbol, N. (2002) *Handboek ter onderbouwing van het verpleegkundig handelen*, 2nd edn. Kavanah, Dwingeloo.

Argyris, C. and Schön, D.A. (1974) *Theory in Practice: Increasing Professional Effectiveness*. Jossey Bass, Washington, DC.

Atkins, S. and Murphy, K. (1993) Reflection: a review of the literature. *Journal of Advanced Nursing*, 18, 1188–92.

Benammar, K. (2004) *Inleiding*. Eindrapport Kenniskring reflectie op het handelen. Hogeschool van Amsterdam, Amsterdam.

Benner, P. (1984) *From Novice to Expert: Uncovering the Knowledge Embedded in Clinical Practice*. Addison-Wesley, Menlo Park, CA.

Bevis, E. (1989) *Curriculum Revolution: Reconceptualizing Nursing Education*. National League for Nursing Press, New York.

Bevis, E. and Watson, J. (1989) *Toward a Caring Curriculum: A New Pedagogy for Nursing*. National League for Nursing Press, New York.

Boyd, E.M. and Fales, A.W. (1983) Reflective learning key to learning from experience. *Journal of Humanistic Psychology*, 23(2), 99–117.

Boykin, A. and Schoenhofer, S. (2001) *Nursing as Caring: A Model for Transforming Practice*. National League for Nursing Press, New York.

Branch, M. and Anderson, M. (1999) Storytelling as a teaching–learning tool with RN students. *Journal of ABNF*, 10(6), 131–5.

Carper, B.A. (1978) Fundamental patterns of knowing in nursing. *Advances in Nursing Science*, 1(1), 13–23.

Cherniss, C. and Goleman, D. (eds) (2001) *The Emotionally Intelligent Workplace: How to select for, measure, and improve emotional intelligence in individuals, groups, and organizations*. Jossey-Bass, San Francisco.

Chinn, P. and Watson, J. (1994) *Art and Aesthetics in Nursing*. National League for Nursing Press, New York.

Clare (1991) Teaching and learning in nurse education: A critical approach. Unpublished PhD thesis, Massey University, Palmerston North, New Zealand.

Clarke, M. (1986) Action and reflection: practice and theory in nursing. *Journal of Advanced Nursing*, 11(1), 3–11.

Clinton, M. (1998) On reflection in action: unaddressed issues in refocusing the debate on reflective practice. *International Journal of Nursing Practice*, 4, 197–202.

Cohen, M., Headley, J. and Sherwood, G. (2000) Spirituality and bone marrow transplantation: When faith is stronger than fear. *International Journal for Human Caring*, 4(2), 41–8.

Cox, H. (1990) Exploring clinical practice: a journey into critical reflection. Unpublished paper presented at the conference: *Embodiment, Empowerment and Emancipation*, Melbourne, Australia.

Cox, H. and Moss, C. (1988) Promiscuous knowledge: the chaos of practice. Conference Proceedings of *Professional Promiscuity*. Olive Anstey Foundation, Perth, Western Australia.

Cox, H., Hickson, P. and Taylor, B. (1991) Exploring reflection: knowing and constructing the practice of nursing, in Gray, G. and Pratt, R. (eds) *Towards a Discipline of Nursing*. Churchill Livingstone, London, 373–89.

Cranton, P. (1996) *Professional Development as Transformative Learning: New Perspectives for Teachers of Adults*. Jossey-Bass, San Francisco.

Croke, E. (2004) The use of structured reflective journal questions to promote fundamental development of clinical decision-making abilities of the first semester nursing student. *Contemporary Nursing*, 17(1–2), 145–36.

Cronenwett, L., Sherwood, G., Barnsteiner, J., Disch, J., Johnson, J., Mitchell, P., Sullivan, D.T. and Warren, J. (2007) Quality and safety education for nurses. *Nursing Outlook*, 55(3), 122–31.

Day, L. and Smith, E. (2007) Integrating quality and safety content into clinical teaching in acute care settings. *Nursing Outlook*, 55(3), 138–43.

Dixon (1996) Critical case studies as voice: The difference in practice between enrolled and registered nurses. Unpublished PhD thesis, Flinders University, Adelaide, Australia.

Dossey, B., Keegan, L. and Guzzetta, C. (2000) *Holistic Nursing: A Handbook for Practice*. Aspen, Gaithersburg, MD.

Drevdahl, D., Stackman, R., Purdy, J. and Louie, B. (2002) Merging reflective inquiry and self-study as a framework for enhancing the scholarship of teaching. *Journal of Nursing Education*, 41(9), 413–19.

Emden, C. (1991) Becoming a reflective practitioner, in Gray, G. and Pratt, R. (eds) *Towards a Discipline of Nursing*. Churchill Livingstone, Melbourne, 335–54.

Esterhuizen, P. (2002) *Morele besluitvorming voor verpleegkundigen*. Bohn Stafleu Van Loghum, Houten.

Forneris, S. and Peden-McAlpine, C. (2007) Evaluation of a reflective learning intervention to improve critical thinking in novice nurses. *Journal of Advanced Nursing*, 57(4), 410–21.

Freshwater, D. (1998) The Philosopher's Stone, in Johns, C. and Freshwater, D. (eds) *Transforming Nursing through Reflective Practice*. Blackwell Publishing, Oxford.

Freshwater, D. and Rolfe, G. (2001) Critical reflexivity: a politically and ethically engaged method for nursing. *NT Research*, 6(1), 526–37.

Freshwater, D. and Rolfe, G. (2004) *Deconstructing Evidence Based Practice*. Taylor & Francis, London.

Ghaye, T. and Ghaye, K. (1998) *Teaching and Learning through Critical Reflective Practice*. David Fullon Publications, London.

Gray, G. and Pratt, R. (eds) (1989) *Issues in Australian Nursing 2*. Churchill Livingstone, Melbourne, Australia.

Gray, G. and Pratt, R. (eds) (1991) *Towards a Discipline of Nursing*. Churchill Livingstone, Melbourne, Australia.

Gray, G. and Pratt, R. (eds) (1992) *Issues in Australian Nursing 3*. Churchill Livingstone, Melbourne, Australia.

Gray, G. and Pratt, R. (eds) (1995) *Issues in Australian Nursing 4*. Churchill Livingstone, Melbourne, Australia.

Greenwood, J. (1993) Reflective practice: a critique of the work of Argyris and Schön. *Journal of Advanced Nursing*, 18, 1183–7.

Greenwood, J. (1998) The role of reflection in single and double loop learning. *Journal of Advanced Nursing Practice*, 27(5), 1048–53.

Habermas, J. (1973) *Knowledge and Human Interests*. Heinemann, London.

Havens, D., Wood, S. and Leeman, J. (2006) Improving nursing practice and patient care: Building capacity with appreciative inquiry. *Journal of Nursing Administration*, 36(10), 463–70.

Hermann, M. (2006) Technology and reflective practice: The use of online discussion to enhance postconference clinical learning. *Nurse Educator*, 31(5), 190–1.

Hesselink, J. (2004) *Zelfsturing, twijfel en inspiratie*. Eindrapport Kenniskring reflectie op het handelen. Hogeschool van Amsterdam, Amsterdam.

Hickson, P. (1988) Knowledge and action in nursing: a critical approach to the practice world of four nurses. Unpublished MA thesis, Massey University, Palmerston North, New Zealand.

Hickson, P. (1990) The promises of critical theory. A paper presented at the conference on *Embodiment, Empowerment and Emancipation*, Melbourne, Australia. In unit NPR 806: Reflective processes in nursing (1991) Deakin University, Geelong, Australia.

Hilgard, E.R. and Atkinson, R. (1979) *Introduction to Psychology*. Harcourt Brace Jovanovich, New York.

Houston, R. (1995) Evaluating quality nursing care through peer review and reflection: the findings of a qualitative study. *International Journal of Nursing Studies*, 32(2), 162–72.

Horton-Deutsch, S. and Horton, J. (2003) Mindfulness: Overcoming intractable conflict. *Archives of Psychiatric Nursing*, 17(4), 186–93.

Institute of Medicine, Committee on the Quality of Health Care in America (2001) *Crossing the Quality Chasm: A New Health System for the 21st Century*. National Academies Press, Washington, DC.

Institute of Medicine (2003) *Keeping Patients Safe: Transforming the Work Environment of Nurses.* National Academies Press, Washington, DC.

Jensen, S. and Joy, C. (2005) Exploring a model to evaluate levels of reflection in baccalaureate nursing students' journals. *Journal of Nursing Education*, 44(3), 139–42.

Johns, C. (1995) Framing learning through reflection within Carper's fundamental ways of knowing in nursing. *Journal of Advanced Nursing*, 22: 226–34.

Johns (1998) Caring through a reflective lens: giving meaning to being a reflective practitioner. *Nursing Inquiry*, 5, 18–24.

Johns, C. and Freshwater, D. (1998) *Transforming Nursing Through Reflective Practice.* Blackwell Science, Oxford.

Johns, C. and Freshwater, D. (2005) *Transforming Nursing Through Reflective Practice*, 2nd edn. Blackwell Publishing, Oxford.

Keefe, M. and Pesut, D. (2004) Appreciative inquiry and leadership transitions. *Journal of Professional Nursing*, 20(2), 103–9.

Kemmis, S. (1985) Action research and the politics of reflection, in Boud, D., Keogh, R. and Walker, D. (eds) *Reflection: Turning Experience into Learning.* Kogan Page, London, 139–64.

Kennison, M. (2006) The evaluation of students' reflective writing for evidence of critical thinking. *Nurse Education Perspectives*, 27(5), 269–73.

Kessler, P. and Lund, C. (2004) Reflective journaling: developing an online journal for distance education. *Nurse Educator*, 29(1), 20–4.

Koetsenruiter, R., van der Heide, W. and Wit, K. (2001) *Reflectie in de verpleegkundige beroepsuitoefening.* Lemma, Utrecht.

Langford, G. (1973) *Human Action*, Doubleday, New York.

Leininger, M. (1978) *Transcultural Nursing: Concepts, Theories, Research and Practice.* McGraw-Hill, New York.

Levett-Jones, T. (2007) Facilitating reflective practice and self-assessment of competence through the use of narratives. *Nurse Education in Practice*, 7, 112–19.

Lumby, J. (1991) *Nursing: Reflecting on an Evolving Practice.* Deakin University Press, Geelong, Australia.

Marcus, M., Liehr, P., Schmitz, J., Moeller, F., Swank, P., Fine, M., Cron, S., Granmayeh, L. and Carroll, D. (2007) Behavioral therapies trials: A case example. *Nursing Research*, 56(3), 210–16.

McCaugherty, D. (1991) The theory–practice gap in nurse education: its causes and possible solutions. Findings from an action research study. *Journal of Advanced Nursing*, 16, 1055–61.

Mensink, F. (1996) Transfer van kennis en ervaring in verpleegkunde: nieuwe wegen voor de reflectieve docent in de combinatiefunctie docent-praktiserend verpleegkundige. *Onderwijs en gezondheidszorg*, 20(8), 152–9.

Moss, C. (2004) Moral-in-practice: a hermeneutic exploration of nurses' choices-in-action during acts of care. Unpublished PhD thesis, Southern Cross University, Lismore, Australia.

Newman, M. (1986) *Health as Expanding Consciousness*. C.V. Mosby, St. Louis, MO.

Nias, J. (1987) *Seeing Anew: Teachers' Theories of Action*. Deakin University Press, Geelong, Australia.

O-Haver Day, P. and Horton-Deutsch, S. (2004) Using mindfulness-based therapeutic interventions in psychiatric nursing practice. Part 1: Description and empirical support for mindfulness-based interventions. *Archives of Psychiatric Nursing*, 18(5), 164–9.

OLVG (2001) Portfolio handleiding en richtlijnen voor het begeleiden van hbov(duaal) – en 'gilde model' – studenten. Onze Lieve Vrouwe Gasthuis, Amsterdam.

Osbourne, P. (1996) Research in Nursing Education, in Cormack, D.F.S. (eds) *The Research Process in Nursing*. Blackwell Publishing, Oxford.

Palmer, A., Burns, S. and Bulman, C. (1994) Reflective Practice in Nursing. Blackwell Publishing, Oxford.

Parker, M. (1994) The healing art of clay: a workshop for remembering wholeness, in Gaut, D. and Boykin, A. (eds) *Caring as Healing: Renewal Through Hope*. National League for Nursing Press, New York.

Paterson, J. and Zderad, L. (1976) *Humanistic Nursing*. National League for Nursing Press, New York.

Peerson, A. and Yong, V. (2003) Reflexivity in nursing: Where is the patient? Where is the nurse? *Australian Journal of Holistic Nursing*, 10(1), 30–45.

Peplau, H. (1952) *Interpersonal Relations in Nursing: A conceptual frame of reference for psychodynamic nursing*. Putnam, New York.

Perry, J. (1985) Theory and practice in the induction of five graduate nurses: a reflexive critique. Unpublished MA thesis, Massey University, Palmerston North, New Zealand.

Perry, J. and Moss, C. (1988) Generating alternatives in nursing: turning curriculum into a living process. *Australian Journal of Advanced Nursing*, 10(4), 1–4.

Powell, J.H. (1989) The reflective practitioner in nursing. *Journal of Advanced Nursing*, 14(10), 824–32.

Richardson, G. and Maltby, H. (1995) Reflection-on-practice: enhancing student learning. *Journal of Advanced Nursing*, 22(2), 235–42.

Rolfe, G. (1998) The theory–practice gap in nursing: from research-based practice to practitioner-based research. *Journal of Advanced Nursing*, 28(3), 672–9.

Rolfe, G., Freshwater, D. and Jasper, M. (2001) *Critical Reflection for Nurses and the Caring Professions: A User's Guide*. Palgrave, Basingstoke.

Ruland, J. and Ahern, N. (2007) Transforming student perspectives through reflective writing. *Nurse Educator*, 32(2), 81–8.

Ruth-Sahd, L. (2003) Reflective practice: a critical analysis of data-based studies and implications for nursing education. *Journal of Nursing Education*, 42(11), 488–97.

Sakalys, J. (2003) Restoring the patient's voice: The therapeutics of illness narratives. *Journal of Holistic Nursing*, 21(3), 228–41.

Schön, D. (1983) *The Reflective Practitioner: How Practitioners Think in Action.* Basic Books, New York.

Sherwood, G. (1997) Developing spiritual care: the search for self, in Roach, S., Sr (ed.) *Caring from the Heart.* Paulist Press, Wahmak, NJ, 196–211.

Sherwood, G. (2000) The power of nurse–client encounter: interpreting spiritual themes. *Journal of Holistic Nursing,* 18(2), 159–75.

Sherwood, G. and Drenkard, K. (2007) Quality and safety curricula in nursing education: matching practice realities. *Nursing Outlook,* 55(3), 151–5.

Smyth, W.J. (1987) *A rationale for teachers' critical pedagogy: A handbook.* Deakin University Press, Geelong, Australia.

Smyth, J. (1992) Teachers' work and the politics of reflection. *American Education Research Journal,* 29(2), 267–300.

Span, P. (1987) Onderwijspsychologie, in Lagerwey, N.A.J. and Vos, J.F., *Onderwijskunde, een inleiding.* Wolters-Noordhoff, Groningen, Netherlands.

Street, A. (1989) Thinking, acting, reflecting: a critical ethnography of clinical nursing practice. Unpublished PhD thesis, Deakin University, Geelong, Australia.

Street, A. (1990) *Nursing Practice: high hard ground, messy swamps and the pathways in between.* Deakin University Press, Geelong, Australia.

Street, A. (1991) *From Image to Action: Reflection in Nursing Practice.* Deakin University Press, Geelong, Australia.

Street, A. (1992) Inside nursing: a critical ethnography of clinical nursing. State University of New York Press, New York.

Strijbol, N. (1996) *In het licht van zorg.* Unpublished Master's dissertation. Utrecht University, the Netherlands.

Swanson, K. (1991) Empirical development of a middle range theory of caring. *Nursing Research,* 40(3), 161–6.

Taylor, B.J. (1997) Big battles for small gains: a cautionary note for teaching reflective processes in nursing and midwifery. *Nursing Inquiry,* 4, 19–26.

Taylor, B.J. (2001) Identifying and transforming dysfunctional nurse–nurse relationships through reflective practice and action research. *International Journal of Nursing Practice,* 7(6), 406–13.

Taylor, B.J. (2002) Becoming a reflective nurse or midwife: using complementary therapies while practising holistically. *Complementary Therapies in Nursing and Midwifery,* 8(4), 62–8.

Taylor, B.J. (2003) Emancipatory reflective practice for overcoming complexities and constraints in holistic health care. *Sacred Space,* 4(2), 40–5.

Taylor, B.J. (2004) Technical, practical and emancipatory reflection for practising holistically. *Journal of Holistic Nursing,* 22(1), 73–84.

Taylor, B.J. (2006) *Reflective Practice: A Guide for Nurses and Midwives,* 2nd edn. Open University Press, Milton Keynes, UK.

Taylor, B.J., Bulmer, B., Hill, L., Luxford, C., McFarlane, J. and Stirling, K. (2002) Exploring idealism in palliative nursing care through reflective practice and action research. *International Journal of Palliative Nursing*, 8(7), 324–30.

Taylor, B., Edwards, P., Holroyd, B., Unwin, A. and Rowley, J. (2005) Assertiveness in nursing practice: an action research and reflection project. *Contemporary Nurse*, 20(2), 324–47.

Teekman, B. (2000) Exploring reflective thinking in nursing practice. *Journal of Advanced Nursing*, 31(5), 1125–35.

Tripp, D. (1987) *Theorising Practice: The Teacher's Professional Journal*. Deakin University Press, Geelong, Australia.

Usher, K. and Holmes, C. (2006) Reflective practice: what, why and how, in Daly, J., Speedy, S. and Jackson, D., *Contexts of Nursing: An Introduction*. Churchill Livingstone, Sydney, Australia, 99–113.

Van de Wiel, H. and Woude, J. (2000) *Zelfzorg voor verpleegkundigen*. Bohn Stafleu Van Loghum, Houten.

Van Parreren, C.F. (1987) Het mensbeeld in de Sovjet-psychologie, in Van Parreren, C.F. and van der Bend, B.J.G., *Psychologie en Mensbeeld*. Ambo, Baarn.

Venneman, B. and Arends, M. (2001) Door vragen wordt men wijs: De reflectievepraktijkvoering. Een model ter bevordering van de eigen methodiekontwikkeling. *Sociale psychiatrie*, 62, 7–14.

Vermunt, J.D.H.M. (1992) Leevstijlen en Sturen van Leerprocessen in het hoger onderwijs [learning styles and guidance of learning processes in higher education]. Suets and Zeitlinger, Amsterdam.

Vitello-Cicciu, J.M. (2002) Exploring emotional intelligence: implications for nursing leaders. *Journal of Nursing Administration*, 32(4), 203–10.

Watson, J. (1979) *Nursing: The Philosophy and Science of Care*. Little Brown, Boston, MA.

Watson, J. (1981) Nursing's scientific quest. *Nursing Outlook*, 29(7), 413–16.

Wellard, S. and Street, A.F. (1999) Family issues in home-based care. *International Journal of Nursing Practice*, 5, 132–6.

Part II

Developing, leading and managing practice through reflection

Chapter 5

Using critical reflection to improve practice

Philip Esterhuizen and Dawn Freshwater

Introduction

A generally held belief relating to reflection is that it leads to aware-ness which in turn can lead to practice improvement (Becker Hentz and Lauterbach, 2005; Driscoll, 2000; Noveletsky-Rosenthal and Solomon, 2001). This can be seen fundamentally as an educationalist perspective to empowerment and emancipation, referred to through-out this text. Bruner (1996: 19) for example suggests that:

> *'thinking about thinking' has to be a principal ingredient of any empowering practice of education.*

This statement, though seemingly quite simple and obvious, camou-flages a complex picture, which suggests that reflection is primarily an educational tool. We believe this requires some further analysis and explanation. Hence, this chapter focuses on the role of reflection and reflective practice in relation to clinical practice; and examines the concepts of critical reflection and guided reflection as ways of improv-ing clinical practice and supporting collaborative research. Assuming an underlying premise that reflective practice is a way of being – that is to say, an embodied ideology – within the confines of this chapter reflection is generally referred to as taking place within structured sessions for nursing students and registered healthcare practitioners.

Reflection as an educational intervention

As outlined in previous chapters, nursing literature over the years (Johns, 2002; Johns and Freshwater, 1998, 2005; Taylor, 2000) has highlighted, and still does, the importance and benefits of reflection and the value of being a reflective practitioner. Several authors have written about reflection and reflective practice as being a transformational tool both for the individual and for nursing practice (Johns and Freshwater, 2005; McCormack and Henderson, 2007).

Nevertheless the way in which healthcare practitioners view and apply reflection and reflective practice is variable. This begs the question: how does one establish a culture within the clinical or academic settings to support reflection and reflective practice?

Although beneficial, establishing a culture that develops reflection and reflective practice can prove a challenge when faced with the perceived pressure of work and time constraints as experienced by healthcare professionals. Time for reflection is often not seen as work in a conventional sense and is often viewed, paradoxically, as being divorced from direct patient care. Consequently, setting time aside for reflective sessions is low on the priority list of those working in the clinical setting. Individuals may consider themselves to have limited resources available, or they may envisage themselves as being individualists within their group of colleagues and, therefore, not needing to take part in group reflection. They are, however, bound to their roles by symbols in their interactions with others in their group (of colleagues) and their environment (Berger and Luckman, 1966; Cohen, 1985). Although it is important to reflect on situations personally, it is essential to also have facilitated reflection and dialog in order for the individual to become aware of their thinking and rationale, and allow them to be confronted with ideas of others in order to develop professional boundaries and identity (Cox, 2005; Day, 1993; Johns, 1994a). We should also remain aware that we all use methods of interaction, reflection and reflexivity to understand and adapt to our environment and that the interaction between facilitator and individual or group is, in itself, part of the awareness, understanding and adaptation process.

Although reflection and reflective practice have been spoken about for numerous decades many healthcare professionals are still skeptical about the value of reflection and are reticent to become involved. This may on occasion be representative of the level of knowledge and understanding of what reflection is, how it can be used, the practical and philosophical application of reflection and of course prior experience of reflection and reflective practice in the clinical and academic settings (Glaze, 2002; Wellard and Bethune, 1996). To some degree this is illustrated in the way Cox (2005) discusses the difference between those individuals using reflection from working in practice as part of a specific program and those developing and learning from their work experience in general. It would appear that learning through reflecting on work situations occurs more readily when it is within the framework of a structured program and linked to specific and prescribed goals or outcomes.

Cox's (2005) work is substantiated by the notion that, among some staff, there is an element of their questioning the need to reflect on the philosophical aspects of their profession, while they may appear more open to exploring practical, patient-related issues of care (Glaze, 2002; Palmer *et al.*, 1994). The work of these authors resonates with our own observations. It would seem that an individual's involvement in reflective sessions seems to create feelings of anxiety and vulnerability that they will be exposed in some way or another when teasing out specific situations they have encountered. (This is particularly interesting when viewed from both an intrapersonal and interpersonal perspective on the self, and is developed further in Chapter 8.) However, having said that, experienced staff members appear more able to reflect on their own position in relation to the other and are less likely to want to explore specific patient-related tasks in any great detail. They seem, rather, to use reflective sessions to validate their actions and ideas.

Similarly many undergraduate student nurses, at the outset, feel that protected time for a reflective session while on a clinical placement is paramount to self-indulgent navel-gazing that keeps them away from the more interesting and exciting world of *real* nursing – working with patients. They identify with the perception that reflective sessions are looking for problems. This attitude generally resolves itself once there has been a difficult or confronting situation with a patient or colleague and the student is able to utilize the reflective session to discuss their experience. The student's (often emotive) input allows them to deconstruct an actual situation rather than discussing what they, until then, had seen to be hypothetical issues and, as a result, are able to see the benefit and value of applying the reflective cycle. This observation links with the work of Johns (2002), where he discusses the phenomenon of practitioners initially feeling that they need to discuss negative experiences during reflective sessions. It is only with time that the individual progresses to use a reflective session as a means of validation and self-exploration. Cox (2005) also discusses the idea of staff members who learn from their work experience viewing reflection as *looking for problems* – this could suggest the importance of facilitated reflection, but also illustrates the difficulty of motivating individuals to engage in reflection in order to develop at a personal level when specific program goals and set objectives are absent.

The undergraduate's attitude to reflection and reflective sessions can also indicate a propensity to focus on tasks and activities, rather than recognizing the contextuality of the situation as described by Benner (1984), and may also be influenced by the (negative) attitudes and opinions of the registered staff they work with (Farrell, 2001; Freshwater, 2000; Philpin, 1999; Randle, 2003).

In Esterhuizen's (2007) recent research with undergraduate students there appeared to be a marked difference in how reflection was viewed and its benefit as they moved through their four-year program. One student commented that as a result of interviews:

> *By talking about things and not only thinking I can move on with things and break the circle. I learn from writing critical incident reports and from talking with you – this is also a sort of reflection. That way I move on with my thinking, otherwise I just stay in a circle.* (Esterhuizen, 2007: 111)

A second respondent, Olga, used peer experiences as an active part of her learning process. She maintained that listening to the reflections of others led her to learn from the situation, but it also allowed her to project the benefit of learning from others into the future with regard to understanding reactions and attitudes. This vicarious learning is a direct outcome of guided group reflection. This student refers to the benefits of guided reflection by discussing the problems she had with using a structured template for reflection and critical incident analysis – she found it restrictive to work with a predefined framework and unhelpful in analyzing the situations she encountered in practice (Esterhuizen, 2007: 86).

If we are then to apply reflection to our work as researchers or facilitators of reflection, we need to be mindful of how we use reflective methods with staff and students. Equally important, we need to be reflexive when supporting nurses to find their own methods of applying reflection to practice, rather than attempting to teach reflective skills by a rote learning method.

Critical reflection and guided reflection

It is easy use the terms reflection and reflective practice rather glibly, mainly because they have been part of the nursing vocabulary for many years. But when we look at the process of guiding an individual through applying the reflective cycle it becomes clear that it is a complex and often confronting exercise that requires facilitation. While it may be true that all individuals have the human ability to reflect, they often need to be supported and facilitated to structure their reflections, remain focussed, and develop skills that allow them to extend their boundaries. This is the role of a facilitator in guided reflection (McCormack and Henderson, 2007; Williams and Walker, 2003).

While the use of models and cues may be helpful in familiarizing individuals with reflection, reflective practice and reflexivity, they also carry a potential risk. By theorizing reflection we run the risk of alienating practitioners who either are not familiar with reflection and reflective practice in a professional sense or see a reflective session as yet another activity removing them from the patient's bedside. We should not lose sight of the fact that reflection is a natural process we continually apply to create order in our lives and understand our life experiences.

One could argue that we should be content to use the term *reflection* rather than *critical reflection* in our discussion as one could say that to reflect is to be human – without reflection we would be unable to function in the social roles we have or within the groups we are part of (Berger and Luckman, 1966; Carrithers, 1992; Cohen, 1985). To return to Chapter 1, in which critical reflection was outlined and defined in relation to reflection and reflexivity, we contend that as the individual reflects on issues, this process will always include an inherent element of critique. It could be argued then that at one level the critical nature of reflection is related to whether the individual uses the reflective process to actively learn in order to apply the insights they gain to future activities.

However, at another level *critical* reflection refers to the depth at which the individual reflects on themselves in relation to a given situation or phenomenon, namely, the degree to which the individual can move from reflecting solely on their actions to reflect on the thought processes driving their actions (Freshwater, 2007; Morley, 2007). Although Morley (2007) and Freshwater (2007) appear to frame their ideas of critical reflection in slightly different terms, both are concerned with how the individual positions themselves in relation to that which they are reflecting on.

Morley (2007) suggests that critical reflection allows the individual to *challenge internal boundaries* in order to liberate themselves from the perceived constructs that limit their actions and thoughts. By using critical reflection, the individual becomes aware of their assumptions and position within the context and discourse of the social structure of which they are a part. The individual's new awareness allows them to reframe their perception of the environment and question their own position in order to improve practice. Freshwater (2007: 56) argues that reflection (thinking about practice) and critical reflection (thinking about thinking, while thinking about practice) are not to be seen in comparative or hierarchical terms, but are essential components for reflexivity (a meta-reflection challenging assumptions in order to gain new awareness). Both authors postulate critical reflection as being an essential component to changing practice due to the individual challenging their paradigms of thought and reformulating their ideas due to a new awareness and, as a result, changing their behavior.

Fish (1998) and Lingsma and Scholten (2001) describe the individual's depth of awareness in terms of an iceberg in which only the *doing* is visible above the level of *experience*. At levels deeper to the practical experience are aspects such as thinking and values (see Fig. 5.1).

Fish (1998) and Lingsma and Scholten (2001) argue that by reflecting at depth on practicalities the individual can access deeper levels of awareness which then directly or indirectly affect their practice. A new awareness or the idea of an altered way of thinking can be seen as being transformational for the individual as this indicates a lasting change in their approach and attitude. Lingsma and Scholten (2001)

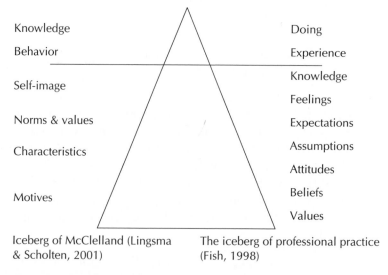

Knowledge		Doing
Behavior		Experience
Self-image		Knowledge
		Feelings
Norms & values		Expectations
Characteristics		Assumptions
		Attitudes
Motives		Beliefs
		Values

Iceberg of McClelland (Lingsma & Scholten, 2001)   The iceberg of professional practice (Fish, 1998)

Figure 5.1 Comparison of depth of awareness: (left) Fish (1998: 99) and (right) Lingsma and Scholten (2001: 55).

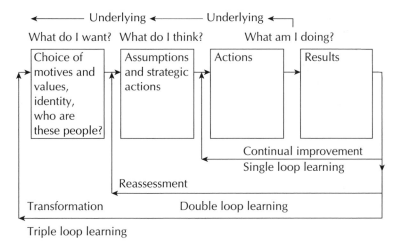

Figure 5.2 Transformational learning (Lingsma and Scholten, 2001: 55).

identify three levels influencing learning: (a) learning from action, (b) learning from becoming aware of assumptions and (c) learning to feel in control of the situation and making choices. They go on to illustrate transformational learning in terms of single, double and triple loop learning (see Fig. 5.2) and suggest that the degree with which the three loops of learning are connected contributes to the degree of permanent change in the individual's development. Each level of learning, therefore, influences those above.

The discussion on transformational learning serves to substantiate the idea of reflection being an educational strategy in the broadest sense and links with Bruner's work (1996) suggesting that this method of learning is, potentially, emancipatory and empowering. It also implies the importance of facilitation and dialog within the reflective process to ensure a progression of depth and focus.

After viewing the literature and reflecting on experience we may acknowledge that reflection is beneficial when used appropriately, but the question still remains as to how reflective practice can be implemented and introduced to practitioners or students who may (initially) be uncertain as to its advantage.

The practicality of reflective models

Implementing reflection in either an academic or a clinical practice arena is a complex and delicate (learning) process which needs to be

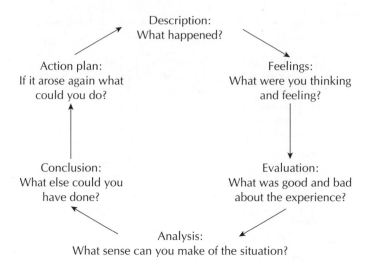

Figure 5.3 Gibbs' reflective cycle (Gibbs, 1988).

understood, addressed with care and nurtured if it is to take root and flourish. As already mentioned, although models of reflection have their place we believe, like their authors, that they should be used as instruments to help reflection and not be prescriptive. As facilitators of reflection, we should take care in meeting the individual's needs and not expect too much too soon. Developing reflective expertise is a complex skill and will develop according to the individual's ability and life experience. When comparing different models of the reflective cycle, although similar in essence, there is a development in the depth and complexity of the cues they provide.

In the Gibbs (1988) model as cited by Johns (2000), although circular, there is an almost linear format to the reflective cycle (see Fig. 5.3) which is descriptive in nature and challenges the individual, through analyzing the situation, to articulate how they make sense of the situation they have encountered.

Driscoll (2000) takes the reflective cycle a step further by augmenting it with 'What?' questions at intervals throughout – 'What?' a description of the event; 'So what?' an analysis of the event; and 'Now what?' proposed actions following the event (see Fig. 5.4). While, as Driscoll (2000) suggests, the 'What' model of reflection is not intended to prescribe a format, it does offer a pragmatic structure to enter into a focussed exploration in all stages of the reflective cycle.

The Gibbs (1988) and Driscoll (2000) models of the reflective cycle provide practitioners with a systematic application of reflection to

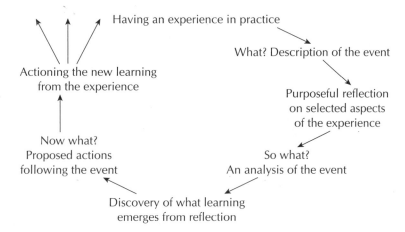

Figure 5.4 'What?' model of structured reflection (Driscoll, 2000).

practice which allows them to answer the questions that arise from the practicalities of their daily work.

When we speak of improving practice we think immediately of the patient and how healthcare practitioners can improve their experience. In Johns' (1994b) original work on reflection, he focussed his reflective cues on what information the nurse needed in order to nurse their patient (Box 5.1). These are practical cues that support the health practitioner to meet their client's needs and identify their personal role in caring for the individual.

Johns (2002) goes on to develop his system of cues (Box 5.2), but appears to move away from viewing only the patient's needs to include the environment and internal world of the healthcare practitioner.

Box 5.1 Burford NDU model: caring in practice (Johns, 1994a).

- Who is this person?
- What health event brings them into hospital?
- How must this person be feeling?
- How has this event affected their usual life patterns and roles?
- How does this person make me feel?
- How can I help this person?
- What is important for this person to make their stay in hospital comfortable?
- What support does this person have in life?
- How do they view the future for themselves and others?

Box 5.2 Model for structured reflection (Johns, 2002).

- Bring the mind home.
- Write a description of an experience that seems significant in some way.
- What issue seemed significant to pay attention to?
- How was I feeling and what made me feel that way?
- What was I trying to achieve?
- Did I respond effectively and in tune with my values?
- What were the consequences of my actions on the patient, others and myself?
- How were others feeling?
- What made them feel that way?
- What factors influenced the way I was feeling, thinking or responding?
- What knowledge did or might have informed me?
- To what extent did I act for the best?
- How does this situation connect with previous experiences?
- How might I respond more effectively given this situation again?
- What would be the consequences of alternative actions for this patient, others and myself?
- How do I feel about this experience?
- Am I now more able to support myself and others better as a consequence?
- Am I more available to work with patients/families and staff to help them meet their needs?

In Johns' most recent work (2006) he suggests that reflective consciousness can be developed further to include abstractions such as energy fields, world philosophy and the cosmos. This ontological approach resonates strongly with ideas previously postulated by Watson (1988), Taylor (1994), Boykin and Schoenhofer (2001) and Nåden and Eriksson (2000, 2002, 2004) in which spiritual consciousness and humanness underpin care and understanding. While personal reflection in relation to a far broader perspective may be essential, it does pose challenges to facilitators involved in developing reflective practice. How does one engage practitioners involved at a practical level to reflect at a deeper, personal level when they often appear to have set themselves boundaries in an attempt to separate professional and personal identities? Whilst we appreciate that any separation of identities could not be feasible from a holistic perspective, this is often the reality facing facilitators when initiating reflection into the clinical setting. Collaborative research with practitioners into their reflective experience is, therefore, vital in understanding the process of developing as a reflective practitioner.

Research and reflective practice

From a small selection of available research publications we can see that practitioners' reflective experiences are being mapped and vary from practical applications of reflective models to complex philosophical discussions.

For example, Hobbs (2007) and Noveletsky-Rosenthal and Solomon (2001) discuss the applicability of Johns' reflective model. Hobbs (2007) shares the deep understanding and communication between a nursing student and his patients that was uncovered by guided reflection. In this instance the author describes her own journey to consciously use Johns' work on reflective practice to understand her own position in relation to the other and recognizes the importance of engaging – failure to engage would result in suffering for the patient and the practitioner.

And in their work with nurse-practitioners Noveletsky-Rosenthal and Solomon (2001) discuss how they use Johns' model for structured reflection to retrospectively analyze clinical situations. In this context Johns' reflective model is not simply applied as an educational tool in isolation, but is situated within Newman's concept of consciousness (Newman, 1994). It is this application of a reflective model within the framework of a philosophy that makes it a powerful educational instrument.

The application of Johns' model as described by the previous authors can be paralleled with the work by Nåden and Eriksson (2000) who discuss nursing as being an art and their research describes components of an *aesthetic encounter* during which the healthcare practitioner clearly applies reflective cues similar to those later described by Johns (2002). In Nåden and Eriksson's (2000) work this is not a retrospective deconstruction of reality, but a spontaneous and embodied interaction between humans based on communicative and linguistic competence. Nåden and Eriksson maintain that the successful application of these competencies is directly related to the ideology of the institution offering the education. They suggest that the practitioner engages with the patient by embodying the communicative competencies they have learned through the ideology they have been exposed to in their education, and differentiate between learned behavior (external confirmation) and living an ideology (internal confirmation). Nåden and Eriksson (2000: 26) quote a nurse in their research as saying:

> *It's about accepting the other person one hundred percent, with all the things he brings along. In these moments I feel that I'm in contact with the deepest of myself.*

Although there is no explicit reference in this work by Nåden and Eriksson to the use of reflective models per se, again embodied reflective practice is placed within a philosophical framework. In this case, the educational ideology is based on Eriksson's notion of caring which incorporates reflection and reflexivity as core concepts (Eriksson, 1997).

Dialogic interaction during reflective sessions has the potential to uncover emotive and sometimes traumatic experiences and the facilitator needs to be mindful of what this may mean to the individual. Morley (2007) discusses her experiences with healthcare practitioners and their feelings of powerlessness in relation to their position. Unless the facilitator is aware of the practitioner's situation, reflection and the subsequent awareness for the individual could result in disempowerment rather than emancipation. However, we feel that it would be paternalistic to assume that practitioners engaging in reflective sessions are always victims of the situation and passive followers of where the facilitator leads. In Esterhuizen's study into the professional socialisation of student nurses:

> *'(retrospective) reflection with mentor, family or partner provide the biggest learning curve', 'I talk informally with the team, mentor and educator about my boundaries – it provides insight'* (Esterhuizen, 2007: 78).

Another student in the same research project, identified as Marijke, returned after an extended period of illness following surgery and spoke of how the educator insisted she formulate learning goals and objectives. Marijke found this approach difficult to understand, but explained how reflective sessions in the classroom setting helped her to develop insight. She tells of how, during the placement on the previous ward, she took her reflections to a deeper level. This deeper reflective level was one of professional growth and development that provided her with a sense of peace (Esterhuizen, 2007: 142).

There are many accounts of research incorporating aspects of reflection and reflective practice (for example, Becker Hentz and Lauterbach, 2005; Cave and Clandinin, 2007; Nåden and Eriksson, 2000, 2002, 2004; Noveletsky-Rosenthal and Solomon, 2001; Spouse, 2003), and the narrative nature of reflection provides a vast amount of data for potential research. It is important to position the information shared by those individuals participating in reflective research. When questioned about her choice of situation to be discussed in a reflective session, one student answered:

> *There are so many important situations and not all situations are discussed during the interviews or reflection. I make a choice.* (Esterhuizen, 2007: 71)

The realization that the individual only ever provides a selection of information surrounding a situation and then packages it as a story with a beginning, a middle and an end and that we, as listeners, create our own story and interpretation must call us to pause and reflect. As facilitators and researchers of reflection and reflective practice it is vital that we strive to increase our understanding of the phenomenon, but we also need to remain realistic in our endeavors to oversimplify the complexity of being human.

Is reflection then a way of improving practice and if it is, how do we measure such an elusive, but expensive commodity?

Reflection as a way of improving practice

So far we have touched briefly on critical and guided reflection and looked at reflection as an educational intervention and the practicality of reflective models. But what does this actually mean for the practitioner and their patients? As previously discussed, reflection and critical thinking have been important developments in nursing education (Johns, 1998; Lyons, 1999; Paul and Heaslip, 1995; Platzer *et al.*, 2000). Jarvis *et al.* (1998) argue that, although reflective learning occurs within a cultural context, they feel that it provides the individual with an abstract approach to learning. As a result they believe that the individual is more comfortable in questioning the status quo of their work environment. This development links with the idea of transformational learning in which the individual develops awareness and insight to critique their daily practice and its organization.

However, to participate in research or to achieve academic credits or professional accreditation, individuals are often required to present their reflective and critical thinking in an assignment or journal format (Glaze, 2002; Hillard, 2006; Lepp *et al.*, 2005; Liimatainen *et al.*, 2001; Noveletsky-Rosenthal and Solomon, 2001; Samuels and Betts, 2007) – a format that, in itself, fuels an ethical debate.

Although not all journals or logs may be assessed, the fact that they are being read *by* others – and perhaps are even being written *for* others – will, by its very nature, alter the content and way it is written. By attempting to develop an assessment system for reflective narrative, it could be said that nursing education is attempting to contain the thoughts of the individual and prescribe the direction of the student's growth (Watson, 2002). At the same time, sharing the content of a very personal, reflective narrative with third parties as a means of assessment or accreditation accentuates the individual's vulnerability (Cotton, 2001). Pryce (2002) takes this argument further by suggesting that deconstruction and analysis of the narrative on the part of the facilitator is undermining to the individual's development. These two approaches dealing with the 'measured' outcomes of reflective practice could result in polarity – one attempting to maintain the status quo and the other stimulating change.

Earlier in the chapter we mentioned the feelings of vulnerability and exposure as experienced by practitioners. This is an important aspect to take into consideration if reflection and reflective practice are, in any way, to contribute to the development of the individual specifically or healthcare practice in general. But how realistic are the individual's feelings of vulnerability? Gilbert (2001) criticizes reflective practice as being a means of surveillance. Within the framework of academic and healthcare provision in which there is an explicit expectation that practitioners reflect and maintain portfolios we could argue that reflective sessions become an institutionalized form of surveillance in which individuals are coerced into sharing their private thoughts and decision-making processes in order to be *corrected* when and if necessary. This is a theme picked up by Freshwater (2005), who writes of the role of surveillance in prison nursing settings and its impact upon the development of reflective practice in those same institutionalized environments. This is contrary to the concept of developing an autonomous practitioner who is able to make judgments and decisions based on their own knowledge and experience. It also implies that one individual has the knowledge and status – with the resultant power – to assess another, bearing in mind that the topics discussed during a reflective session are usually not about the practicalities of practice, but often focus on very private and sensitive issues, fundamental to the individual's being. In the case of group sessions, it is the collective consciousness that *corrects* the individual into adapting to a group norm – the assumption being that this would represent professional opinion, norms and values. This is, of course, one way of thinking about it. Another way could be to view this correction as being oppressive. Much has been published on nurses being an oppressed group and the existence of horizontal violence within the concept of professional socialisation (Farrell, 2001; Freshwater, 2000). Structured reflective sessions facilitated by someone from the same profession and from within the same organization could be interpreted as being the optimal success of an oppressed society in which peers exercise control over each other (Freire, 1970).

The idea of individuals being coerced into writing their reflections according to a prescribed format was reflected in the responses to Esterhuizen's study in which students mention the difficulty they had with the prescribed format, signifying the importance of choice of who they reflected with, when and to what depth. More specifically, the idea of coercion is articulated by Sinclair-Penwarden (2006) when she questions the educational organization's right to request that personal information be shared and consequently graded. Ghaye (2007) uses Sinclair-Penwarden's criticism to discuss the ethics of reflective portfolios and their educational impact. Part of this ethical criticism is around the idea of role-modeling – how can a student be expected to value and respect the privacy of her patient, when her own privacy is being violated? Another part is concerned with the effect this violation will have on her development as a person and an individual. Does an intervention such as a reflective portfolio address her learning needs? Or is this yet another symptom of a voyeuristic society in which the media leaves no stone unturned and exposes viewers and readers to painfully personal experiences? But to what end? Reflection and reflective practice have the potential to be disempowering, damaging and destructive, so how do they improve practice?

What lessons can be learned?

Anecdotes from the literature and from experience indicate that there is a potential polarization for and against reflection and reflective practice. However, it is important to clarify whether the criticism leveled is at reflection and reflective practice as a means of learning and improving practice, or whether it is about the potential abuse of an individual using reflection as a means to an end, namely control.

In our experience, there is no doubt that individuals develop due to guided reflection in which their decisions and choices, influences and assumptions have become conscious and their awareness has influenced the way they have approached similar situations in the future. We view this development in the context of the individual's life experience and any conclusions of personal transformation need be made by the person concerned. In other words, although reflection may be guided and the individual facilitated to view themselves within the context of their environment and/or relationships, the process the individual moves through is fundamentally personal and private. Reflection should not be used as a method for assessing competencies of decision making, ethical awareness or professional development. Pryce (2002) suggests that reflection provides an opportunity for an individual to identify, and perhaps even discover, another facet of their being – a facet just as valid and relevant as any other truths they own – or a new view to complement the meanings they already hold on a situation.

Summary

Facilitating practitioners to understand the world they live and work in; making sense of how the different roles they have can complement each other, rather than vie for supremacy; and understanding their position within social and political arenas are some of the values of critical reflection. But it is also about reflecting and being reflexive as a facilitator: understanding and remaining aware that the issues pertaining to practitioners who participate in reflection are equally pertinent to those of us who facilitate or research – we cannot remove ourselves from the equation. We are part of the process and the only authority we have is to identify what is valid and meaningful for ourselves. Identifying what is meaningful in relation to practice will result in personal awareness and will, ultimately, allow us to deal with situations strategically rather than reactively.

Improvement to practice through reflection, therefore, leads to a conscious, strategic practitioner who is proactive rather than reactive in dealing with patient-related and political situations; one who understands what drives them, not within a coerced method of control, but as an intrinsic, emancipatory force.

References

Becker Hentz, P. and Lauterbach, S.S. (2005) Becoming self-reflective: caring for self and others. *International Journal for Human Caring*, 9(1), 24–8.
Benner, P. (1984) *From Novice to Expert: Excellence and Power in Clinical Nursing Practice*. Addison-Wesley, Menlo Park, CA.

Berger, P. and Luckman, T. (1966) *The Social Construction of Reality: A Treatise in the Sociology of Knowledge.* Penguin, London.

Boykin, A. and Schoenhofer, S.O. (2001) *Nursing as Caring: A Model for Transforming Practice.* Jones & Bartlett, Sudbury, MA (for National League for Nursing).

Bruner, J. (1996) *The Culture of Education.* Harvard University Press, London.

Carrithers, M. (1992) *Why Humans have Cultures: Explaining Anthropology and Social Diversity.* Oxford University Press, Oxford.

Cave, M.T. and Clandinin, D.J. (2007) Learning to live with being a physician. *Reflective Practice*, 8(1), 75–91.

Cohen, A.P. (1985) *The Symbolic Construction of Community.* Routledge, London.

Cotton, A.H. (2001) Private thoughts in public spheres: issues in reflection and reflective practices in nursing. *Journal of Advanced Nursing*, 36(4), 512–19.

Cox, E. (2005) Adult learners learning from experience: using a reflective practice model to support work-based learning. *Reflective Practice*, 6(4), 459–72.

Day, C. (1993) Reflection: a necessary but not sufficient condition for professional development. *British Educational Research Journal*, 19(1), 83–93.

Driscoll, J. (2000) *Practising Clinical Supervision.* Baillière Tindall, London.

Eriksson, K. (1997) Caring, spirituality and suffering, in *Caring from the Heart: The Convergence of Caring and Spirituality.* Paulist Press, New York.

Esterhuizen, P. (2007) The journey from neophyte to registered nurse – a Dutch experience. Unpublished PhD thesis. Bournemouth University, UK.

Farrell, G.A. (2001) From tall poppies to squashed weeds: why don't nurses pull together more? *Journal of Advanced Nursing*, 35(1), 26–33.

Fish, D. (1998) *Appreciating Practice in the Caring Professions: Refocusing Professional Development and Practitioner Research.* Butterworth-Heinemann, Oxford.

Freshwater, D. (2000) Crosscurrents: against cultural narration in nursing. *Journal of Advanced Nursing*, 32(2), 481–4.

Freshwater, D. (2005) Clinical supervision in the context of custodial care, in Freshwater, D. and Johns, C. (eds) *Transforming Nursing through Reflective Practice*, 2nd edn. Blackwell Publishing, Oxford.

Freshwater, D. (2007) Reflective practice and clinical supervision: two sides of the same coin? in Bishop, V. (ed.) *Clinical Supervision*, 2nd edn. Palgrave, Basingstoke, UK.

Freire, P. (1970) *Pedagogy of the Oppressed.* Penguin, London.

Ghaye, T. (2007) Editorial: Is reflective practice ethical? (The case of the reflective portfolio) *Reflective Practice*, 8(2), 151–62.

Gibbs, G. (1988) *Learning by doing: a guide to teaching and learning methods.* Further Education Unit, Oxford Polytechnic, now Oxford Brookes University.

Gilbert, T. (2001) Reflective practice and clinical supervision: meticulous rituals of the confessional. *Journal of Advanced Nursing*, 36(2), 199–205.

Glaze, J.E. (2002) Stages in coming to terms with reflection: student advanced nurse practitioners' perceptions of their reflective journeys. *Journal of Advanced Nursing*, 37(3), 265–72.

Hillard, C. (2006) Using structured reflection on a critical incident to develop a professional portfolio. *Nursing Standard*, 21(2), 35–40.

Hobbs, K. (2007) The power of reflective practice in second-degree nursing education. *International Journal for Human* Caring, 11(1), 22–4.

Jarvis, P., Holford, J. and Griffin, C. (1998) *The Theory and Practice of Learning*. Kogan Page, London.

Johns, C. (1994a) Guided reflection, in Palmer, A., Burns, S. and Bulman, C. (eds) *Reflective Practice in Nursing*. Blackwell Science, Oxford.

Johns, C. (1994b) *The Burford NDU Model: Caring in Practice*. Blackwell Science, Oxford.

Johns, C. (1998) Caring through a reflective lens: giving meaning to being a reflective practitioner. *Nursing Inquiry*, 5, 18–14.

Johns, C. (2000) *Becoming a Reflective Practitioner*. Blackwell Science, Oxford.

Johns, C. (2002) *Guided Reflection: Advancing Practice*. Blackwell Science, Oxford.

Johns, C. (2006) *Engaging Reflection in Practice: A Narrative Approach*. Blackwell Publishing, Oxford.

Johns, C. and Freshwater, D. (1998) *Transforming Nursing Through Reflective Practice*, 1st edn. Blackwell Science, Oxford.

Johns, C. and Freshwater, D. (2005) *Transforming Nursing Through Reflective Practice*, 2nd edn. Blackwell Science, Oxford.

Lepp, M., Zorn, C.R., Duffy, P.R. and Dickson, R.J. (2005) Swedish and American nursing students use journaling for reflection: an international student-centered learning experience. *International Journal for Human Caring*, 9(4), 52–8.

Liimatainen, L., Poskiparta, M., Karhila, P. and Sjögren, A. (2001) The development of reflective learning in the context of health counselling and health promotion during nurse education. *Journal of Advanced Nursing*, 34(5), 648–58.

Lingsma, M. and Scholten, M. (2001) *Coachen op competentieontwikkeling*. Uitgeverij Nelissen, Soest.

Lyons, J. (1999) Reflective education for professional practice: discovering knowledge from experience. *Nurse Education Today*, 19, 29–34.

McCormack, B. and Henderson, L. (2007) Critical reflection and clinical supervision: facilitating transformation, in Bishop, V. (ed.) *Clinical Supervision*, 2nd edn. Palgrave, Basingstoke, UK.

Morley, C. (2007) Engaging practitioners with critical reflection: issues and dilemmas. *Reflective Practice*, 8(1), 61–74.

Nåden, D. and Eriksson, K. (2000) The phenomenon of confirmation: an aspect of nursing as an art. *International Journal for Human Caring*, 4(3), 23–8.

Nåden, D. and Eriksson, K. (2002) Encounter: a fundamental category of nursing as an art. *International Journal for Human Caring*, 6(1), 34–40.

Nåden, D. and Eriksson, K. (2004) Understanding the importance of values and moral attitudes in nursing care in preserving human dignity. *Nursing Science Quarterly*, 17(1), 86–91.

Newman, M.A. (1994) *Health as Expanding Consciousness*, 2nd edn. National League for Nursing, New York.

Noveletsky-Rosenthal, H.T. and Solomon, K. (2001) Reflections on the use of Johns' model of structured reflection in nurse-practitioner education. *International Journal for Human Caring*, 5(2), 21–6.

Palmer, A., Burns, S. and Bulman, C. (1994) *Reflective Practice in Nursing*. Blackwell Science, Oxford.

Paul, R.W. and Heaslip, P. (1995) Critical thinking and intuitive practice. *Journal of Advanced Nursing*, 22, 40–7.

Philpin, S.M. (1999) The impact of 'Project 2000' educational reforms on occupational socialization of nurses: an exploratory study. *Journal of Advanced Nursing*, 29(6), 1326–31.

Platzer, H., Blake, D. and Ashford, D. (2000) An evaluation of process and outcomes from learning through reflective practice groups on a post-registration nursing course. *Journal of Advanced Nursing*, 31(3), 689–95.

Pryce, A. (2002) Refracting Experience: reflection, postmodernity and trans-formations. *Journal of Research in Nursing*, 7(4), 298–310.

Randle, J. (2003) Changes in self-esteem during a 3 year pre-registration Diploma in Higher Education (Nursing) programme. *Journal of Clinical Nursing*, 12(1), 142–3.

Samuels, M. and Betts, J. (2007) Crossing the threshold from description to deconstruction and reconstruction: using self-assessment to deepen reflection. *Reflective Practice*, 8(2), 269–83.

Sinclair-Penwarden, A. (2006) Listen up: we should not be made to disclose our personal feelings in reflection assignments. *Nursing Times*, 102(37), 12.

Spouse, J. (2003) *Professional Learning in Nursing*. Blackwell Publishing, Oxford.

Taylor, B.J. (1994) *Being Human: Ordinariness in Nursing*. Churchill Livingstone, Melbourne.

Taylor, B.J. (2000) *Reflective Practice: A Guide for Nurses and Midwives*. Open University Press, Maidenhead, UK.

Watson, J. (1988) *Nursing: Human Science and Human Care – A Theory of Nursing*. National League for Nursing, New York.

Watson, S. (2002) The use of reflection as an assessment of practice. Can you mark learning contracts? *Nurse Education in Practice*, 2, 150–9.

Wellard, S. and Bethune, E. (1996) Reflective journal writing in nurse education: whose interests does it serve? *Journal of Advanced Nursing*, 24(5), 1077–82.

Williams, B. and Walker, L. (2003) Facilitating perception and imagination in generating change through reflective practice groups. *Nurse Education Today*, 23, 131–7.

Chapter 6

Clinical supervision and reflective practice

Philip Esterhuizen and Dawn Freshwater

Introduction

In this chapter we look at the connection between reflection, clinical supervision and reflective practice and discuss definitions and models for supervision and how these interface with reflection. We undertake an in-depth examination of the options of improving practice through reflection, clinical supervision and reflective practice using information, insights and ideas from practitioners involved in establishing clinical supervision in their respective areas.

It is important to contextualize the discussion on reflection and clinical supervision prior to entering into any depth of debate. The idea of an individual wanting to make sense of the experiences they encounter is the point of departure. This says a lot about our ontological approach to reflection and clinical supervision which is based on the assumption that an individual has an intrinsic desire to develop understanding and awareness. This process is the embodiment of work by Maslow (Boeree, 2006) on self-actualization and Knowles (1980) on dimensions of maturation – key elements of adult learners. Being adult is also a key concept to experiential learning and, as Knowles (1980: 50) suggests:

> *Adults* are *what they have* done.

Thus when discussing reflection and clinical supervision, two activities primarily concerned with personal development, we need to look critically at their relationship within the context of an adult learning from experience and what it is we are attempting to achieve through their implementation.

Reflection, clinical supervision and reflective practice: the eternal triangle?

As the concept of reflection has been discussed elsewhere in more detail (see Chapter 1), at this point we only wish to suggest that, from a nursing perspective, reflection has been defined in different ways. Some definitions incorporate the product and the (often emancipatory) process envisaged by the author (Freshwater, 2007; Johns, 2006; Johns and Freshwater, 1998, 2005) whereas others frame reflection in terms of learning (Boud *et al.*, 2000; Jarvis *et al.*, 2001). One could argue that emancipation is *also* learning; albeit in abstract terms with possibly less conventionally measurable outcomes it can, nevertheless, be seen as learning. So, in an attempt to provide a definition of professional reflection that encompasses, for want of a better word, the *pureness* of the commonsense idea of reflection being the *throwing back from a surface*, we use, in the context of this chapter, the definition by Taylor (2000: 3):

> *Reflection means the throwing back of thoughts and memories, in cognitive acts such as thinking, contemplation, meditation and any other form of attentive consideration, in order to make sense of them, and to make contextually appropriate changes if they are required.*

Let us then turn our thoughts to clinical supervision, which is described by numerous authors as being a structured system of reflection important, primarily, to improve practice (Driscoll, 2000; Fish and Twinn, 1997; Spouse and Redfern, 2000; Van Ooijen, 2003). An area that continues to be debated is that of the facilitation of reflective practice; just as practice cannot be changed in isolation, it is argued that practitioners struggle to objectify their own beliefs, values and actions without the benefit of another perspective. Burton (2000) argues that reflection needs to be guided (as was discussed in the previous chapter), referring to the earlier works of Johns (1996) and Cox *et al.* (1991), she advocates support from a skilled supervisor.

Definitions of clinical supervision abound; clinical supervision could be simply described as a flexible and dynamic structure within which to continuously deconstruct and reconstruct clinical practice. Fundamental to this process of deconstruction and reconstruction are the skills of reflection, critical reflection and reflexivity. In other words clinical supervision and reflective practice are interdependent and inextricably linked through the process of reflection. The Nursing and Midwifery Council (NMC) – the national registering body for nursing in the United Kingdom – has embraced this approach to clinical supervision as being an instrument to improve practice and its importance has been accentuated by including it in official publications (NMC, 2002), as has the UK Department of Health (1993) that defines clinical supervision as:

> *A term to describe a formal process of professional support and learning which enables practitioners to develop knowledge and competence, assume responsibility for their own practice and enhance consumer protection and safety of care in complex situations.*

Bishop (2006: 17) suggests that clinical supervision is:

> *A designated interaction between two or more practitioners within a safe and supportive environment, that enables a continuum of reflective, critical analysis of care, to ensure quality patient services, and the well-being of the practitioner.*

In contrast to the published definitions above, a working definition suggested by a group of experienced practitioners during a training program on clinical supervision after they had critically discussed the evolved definitions (ALG, 2006) reads as:

> *A time-protected interaction between 2 or more professionals in a safe, supportive and confidential environment to discuss, reflect and critically analyse work issues. The aim of clinical support is to encourage self-development and improve work practices.*

Comparing the definitions provides a few interesting points for discussion. The practitioners' definition illustrates their understanding of the limited resources in 'real life,' as they put it, in which they accentuate the need for protected time. This was one of the most important issues raised as being influential in successfully implementing and sustaining clinical supervision within a department. Another element they include in their definition is the focus on discussing *work issues*, to improve practice, but they also articulate the importance of individual development.

A further observation is the fact that both the Department of Health (1993) and Bishop (2006) suggest clinical supervision as *enabling* practitioners to ensure high-quality care. This illuminates two points of discussion.

The first point we wish to highlight is the use of the word *enable*. Espeland and Shanta (2001) discuss the dichotomy of enabling versus empowering and quote Haber *et al.* (1997: 516) as defining enabling as:

> *behaviours by others that perpetuates dependent behaviours.*

This is contrary to the idea of an adult striving for self-actualization and personal development. More specifically it conflicts with authors who consider reflective processes to be transformational for the individual. However, Bishop's (2006) interpretation of *enable* within the context of her definition appears to relate to a process of analysis being enabled, rather than the practitioner – although this is, in itself, a point of discussion. One could ask whether reflection and clinical supervision should not focus on emancipating the practitioner which would, as a result, enable them to analyze their practice critically.

The second point needing to be highlighted can be developed from the discussion on the semantics of *enabling* versus *emancipation* and is the concept of power and control. Gilbert (2001) suggests that clinical supervision can be seen as a form of surveillance in which organizations are able to establish formal structures exercising control (see previous chapter). The definition used by the Department of Health (1993) in which clinical supervision enables the practitioner to *assume responsibility* implies that this is not happening and the idea of surveillance becomes more tangible when the responsibility to establish supervision is delegated to a local level and the reality is that line managers supervise their staff. Although Bishop (2006) appears to suggest *enabling* rather than *empowering* practitioners, she also highlights the organizational influence. She suggests, amongst other things, that a governmental preoccupation with audit and evidence-based practice could move the focus of clinical supervision away from the philosophical development of individual practitioners towards a method of ensuring standards of quality are being met. Within this context Bishop, we feel, underpins the notion of wanting to enable the practitioner to develop a *process* of critical thought in her definition. The idea of enabling a process has a different weight than the Department of Health definition which suggests incapability.

In other aspects, the definition by Bishop (2006) and the one put forward by the practitioners are comparable in their attention to personal development and quality of care. It is interesting how similar the two definitions are considering that Bishop's (2006) definition had not been published at the time of the program and so the practitioners had not been privy to it when they conceived their personal definition for the purpose of the program.

There is, however, another area of debate, namely that of the nomenclature. Numerous practitioners question the relevance of *clinical* supervision and this terminology results in confusion and frustration as it implies that supervisory sessions may only be used to discuss

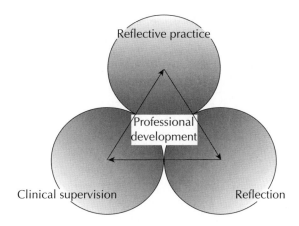

Figure 6.1 Professional development as the common theme between reflective practice, reflection and clinical supervision.

patient-related, clinical issues. In fact many other issues influence the individual practitioner's professional development – not least of all issues relating to management, inter-professional interaction, relationships with peers and patients' families, and organizational concerns.

What then is the connection between clinical supervision, reflection and reflective practice? In our view it is the relationship between reflection and clinical supervision that results in reflective practice (see Fig. 6.1). Where reflection is a cyclic thought process (a skill) and clinical supervision is a method that can be used to focus and guide the individual's reflective process (a structure), the change that arises from this contextualized, analytic process results in reflective practice (a way of being). Driscoll (2000: 21) suggests that:

> *Not all reflective practice is clinical supervision but potentially all good clinical supervision is reflective practice.*

Well-facilitated clinical supervision can provide the cues for reflection allowing the individual to identify their own ways of knowing. In our experience of working with groups, elements of Carper's (1978) patterns of knowing – the science of nursing (empirical), the art of nursing (aesthetics), ethics of care and personal knowledge – are always discussed; initiated by the group members themselves, without too many prompts from the facilitator. Often the practitioners do not categorize or classify their discussion according to Carper's work, but do address the four patterns via the content of their discussion. Insights into our ways of recognizing and understanding the components of our being assist us in being aware of our development and provide footholds towards the elusive concept of self-actualization, or perhaps more specifically, to understand and reach our personal potential in professional development (something that is picked up in Chapter 8).

The areas of reflection, clinical supervision and reflective practice are bound together by a common focus – in this case, the individual's professional development – and, as such, they interrelate. However in some circumstances they can function independently inasmuch that an individual may have internalized elements of their professional role to the degree that they do not need to reflect actively and consciously, as in the case of the expert practitioner (Benner, 1984). In a different situation, the same individual may feel the need to reflect on a specific element of care in order to internalize it and, in yet another situation, they may feel the need for facilitated clinical supervision in order to analyze and understand the implications of a situation, prior to private reflection and incorporation into their scope of practice as a reflective practitioner. When viewed from this perspective, reflection and clinical supervision combine to result in producing a reflective practitioner embodying reflective practice.

Personal development through clinical supervision

When facilitating participants across disciplines in clinical supervision programs it has become apparent that, although the individual's development as a professional is the focus, it does impact on their personal development. It is, therefore, important to keep clinical supervision grounded in their daily work and discipline.

There is a definite tension between accepting and understanding the holistic nature of the individual practitioner, knowing that reflections and awareness in a professional domain will have an impact on their personal life; and accepting and understanding the individual's attempts to maintain a boundary between personal and professional aspects of their life. The diagrammatical representation (Fig. 6.1) in the context of this discussion focusses on professional development but the same principle can, of course, be transferred, by the individual, to other areas of their life.

Although the similarities and differences between clinical supervision and counseling have been discussed by different authors (Bond and Holland, 1998; Driscoll, 2000; Van Ooijen, 2003), it is important to bring these under the reader's attention (Table 6.1).

Because it is impossible for an individual to separate awareness and insight in their professional behavior from impacting on their personal

Table 6.1 Differences between counseling and clinical supervision (Bond and Holland, 1998:134).

	Counseling	Clinical supervision
Agenda	Agenda defined by the supervisee.	Agenda mostly defined by the supervisee. Clinical supervisor may add items arising during the sessions or refocus on how any personal issues discussed affect practice.
Confidentiality	Total, with legal exceptions. Counselor or client may keep own records that are absolutely confidential.	Almost total, with exceptions of legal or professional ethics. Record may be made to pass on within the organization of attendance dates and times. Record of content may be negotiated between practitioner and clinical supervisor, for their eyes only.
Information from facilitator	Information, advice or guidance very rarely given, and then usually focussed on emotional issues.	Some information, advice, guidance offered to supplement the supervisee's own expertise, to help the supervisee see options available and make their own informed decision.
Challenge from facilitator	Non-judgmental about the person's emotional issues. Very occasional challenges about defenses against emotional expression and growth.	Challenging technical mistakes, inadequate clinical standards, and contribution to problems with teamwork, more personal issues such as unhelpful or self-defeating behavior or attitude, blind spots, broken contracts. Based on evidence gained during the clinical supervision session.
Support from facilitator	Support for the client as a person, often especially for emotional awareness and expression. Support is open-ended.	Support for the supervisee as a person and encouragement given to help supervisee recognize and use own expertise and personal abilities towards developing their professional expertise. Any exploration of personal issues eventually related back to how these affect practice. Clinical supervisor acknowledges any emotional issues about the past which are disclosed, but suggests that his/her remit is to help with the present-day feelings and practicalities.
Catalytic help from facilitator	Enabling reflection and problem solving in the direction of deeper exploration into the personal and relationship aspects of the problem, including the transference relationship between client and counselor.	Enabling reflection on issues ultimately affecting practice (including some consideration of issues involved in the clinical supervision relationship), learning from experience, problem solving, pinpointing ways of dealing with difficult emotions, decision making and planning. All of these with the ultimate emphasis on reviewing application to practice.

lives and vice versa, it is important that we remain aware of this phenomenon and maintain a healthy division between (clinical) supervision related to professional issues and counseling on a more personal level. All parties need to be aware that any issue an individual needs to reflect on from a professional perspective generally has a personal component that may need to be addressed. Alternatively, behavior manifesting in a professional setting will often be identified by the individual as occurring in their personal lives too. Realizing and respecting this interface between personal and professional, is the essence of developing self-awareness as an individual in order to adapt behavior and ultimately change or improve practice. However it is imperative that all parties are clear in setting their boundaries.

Driscoll (2000) suggests that while counseling focusses primarily on promoting healing for the client, clinical supervision provides guidance, support and an opportunity to reflect – in a structured way – on a specific, work-related issue. Similarly, Van Ooijen (2003: 45) describes counseling as developing *a greater personal awareness of one's inner landscape*, whereas supervision focusses on work. Both authors are clear that, while being aware of the overlap between counseling and supervision, all parties have the responsibility to identify and maintain clear boundaries when personal issues manifest themselves. The supervisor has the explicit responsibility to maintain their role and both Driscoll and Van Ooijen support the principle that the supervisee should address any specific, personal issue – but in a different setting. As part of their role, the supervisor could suggest where the individual may receive help, but in no way should take on the role of counselor.

Considering how confusing the interface between counseling and supervision can be, one option in maintaining clarity could be to set specific goals for each supervisory session in which the focus of the session is articulated. Proctor (1986) suggests a model that could be beneficial in helping the supervisee set an agenda and maintain the necessary focus (see Fig. 6.2).

While it is clear from Proctor's model that any supervision session will incorporate all three functions, often one is more predominant. Supporting the supervisee to analyze which focus they want supervision to have prior to the session, and evaluating at the end whether this was, in fact, the most appropriate choice, using Proctor's model, could provide the supervisee with a practical, transferable skill of being able to recognize an issue and focus on it during personal reflection. A final consideration while on the subject of personal and professional boundaries is that, while holistic in our approach to the

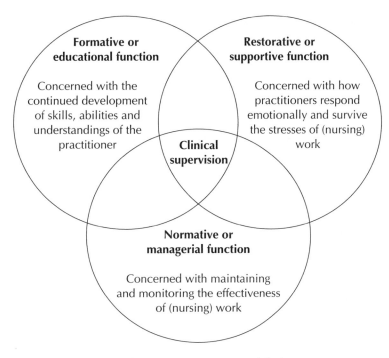

Figure 6.2 Three functions of Proctor's interactive model of supervision.

individual, we would do well to remember that reflection or clinical supervision on professional issues – while important – is *one* part of the larger picture for the individual. Professional investment is but one section of the individual's life and not the other way around. Retaining this principle could also be useful in helping the supervisee maintain perspective on professional situations and be helpful in setting boundaries for both supervisee and supervisor.

The centricity of practice in clinical supervision

Freshwater (2007) refers to the work of Donald Schön (1987) and suggests the importance of reflecting on experience in order to contextualize the situation and therefore learn from it. As we have already indicated with Proctor's work, we too think it is important that a practitioner maintains the focus on practice-related situations during supervision.

Another way of supporting a practitioner to reflect on their clinical role would be to incorporate the four different aspects of their role as a means of approaching and analyzing a practice-related situation they

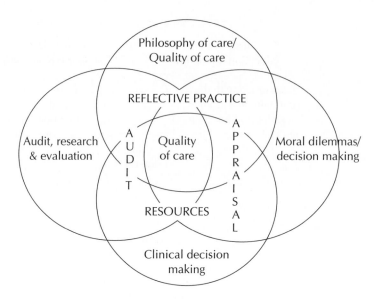

Figure 6.3 Quality of care as the focus of clinical supervision.

wish to discuss during supervision (Fig. 6.3) in which quality of care will, generally, be the driving force behind the choice of topic.

As Fig. 6.3 does not indicate direction in using the four aspects to analyze a situation, a practitioner can approach their analysis from whichever perspective they consider to be the most appropriate or to have the greatest priority. Using this type of approach provides neutrality for the practitioner and, although the discussion focusses on their specific issues, the model allows for structure and a feeling of *objectivity* which may make supervision less threatening to the individual. Linked to Proctor's model, the practitioner is able to identify specific issues needing to be addressed. Clinical supervision sessions focussing on the quality of care can be used equally effectively for individual and group supervision – the latter having the advantage of providing a shared learning experience among colleagues.

Fish and Twinn (1997) discuss two models of clinical supervision which illustrate the dichotomy between clinical supervision as a method to develop reflective qualities on the one hand and a method to develop competencies on the other. They consider the former to incorporate the *artistry* of care, while the latter is skill-related. With regard to the latter, we need to be aware of the organizational implications of clinical supervision. As Gilbert (2001) suggests, clinical supervision could, potentially, be a method of surveillance. However, Clouder and Sellars (2004) suggest that there may be a case for using clinical supervision as a means of surveillance, considering the miscarriage of ethics by professionals in the course of our healthcare history. Organizations are, after all, responsible for the quality of care provided. Even though individual practitioners are responsible for their actions, any negative publicity will be detrimental to the organization.

The implication of providing facilitated supervision is an expensive commodity for an organization and it could be argued that managers should have some idea as to what is being discussed during supervisory sessions, and that practitioners have a responsibility to provide transparency as to what they consider to be the benefits. Clouder and Sellars (2004) suggest that a possible way forward is be to be explicit (rather than implicit) regarding the use of clinical supervision as a means of obtaining information to ensure high-quality care and provide management with specific information. While Northcott (2000) suggests that clinical supervision could be linked to performance management and annual appraisals, Pesut and Herman's (1999) work on clinical reasoning illustrates how patient-related decision making could be incorporated into supervisory sessions.

While we find it hard to support the idea of clinical supervision being used as a method of control and management, many defend this position. Organizing clinical supervision in this way may ensure that the practitioner remains focussed on work-related issues and reduce the risk that supervisory sessions drift into a counseling mode. It is possible however that the two approaches as described by Fish and Twinn (1997) can be complementary. Johns (2001) illustrates the emancipating versus controlling use of clinical supervision and seems to suggest a polarization related to the intention of the supervisor (Fig. 6.4).

Interestingly the discussions related to the intent–emphasis grid, within the groups of practitioners undertaking a program on clinical supervision, focussed more on the potential complementarities of the approaches rather than their polarization.

Van Ooijen (2003) suggests that the practitioner could benefit from supervision by an outsider and a manager. In some ways this is also a weakness if, as Van Ooijen goes on to suggest, this form of managerial supervision is dependent on the relationship between the parties being balanced and affable. The construction of managerial supervision could create complications if some staff chose managerial supervision, whilst others chose to have clinical supervision from an outsider. Although both methods could result in practitioners learning and developing, it is feasible that it could create discrepancies between staff members within a team.

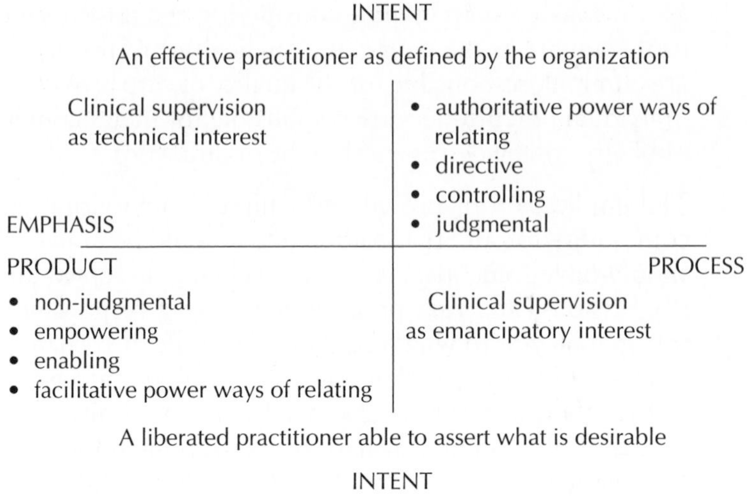

INTENT

An effective practitioner as defined by the organization

Clinical supervision as technical interest	• authoritative power ways of relating • directive • controlling
EMPHASIS	• judgmental

PRODUCT	PROCESS
• non-judgmental • empowering • enabling • facilitative power ways of relating	Clinical supervision as emancipatory interest

A liberated practitioner able to assert what is desirable

INTENT

Figure 6.4 The intent–emphasis grid (Johns, 2001).

The potential difference between managerial and outside facilitation could lie in the terminology – coaching versus clinical supervision. It would be ill-advised to introduce another term for an intervention unless it is clear to all parties what the difference is. Coaching could be undertaken by the unit manager to support individual development towards an agreed point – a team vision/philosophy including specific knowledge and skills (Boud *et al.*, 2000; Scheweer, 2000; Schön, 1987; Spouse and Redfern, 2000) whereas an external facilitator could provide clinical supervision to support personal development. Both coaching and clinical supervision in this context would contribute to personal development, but using specific terminology for specific interventions focussed on achieving particular objectives would provide clarity between the roles.

By creating an opportunity for structured reflection, facilitated by an outsider, and a form of managerial support by way of coaching, it would provide an opening for development and growth on the part of the practitioner, plus the chance for the line manager to meet with their staff and obtain insight as to the development towards achieving objectives as defined by the team.

Discussion

Whilst it would not be true that all the literature around clinical supervision emphasizes the skills of reflection, it is fair to say that the two concepts are often described concurrently. Many models of clinical supervision are presented, nearly all of which include an element of reflection and reflection on practice (Bond and Holland, 1998; Hawkins and Shohet, 1989; Holloway, 1995); others suggest reflection is itself a model for supervision (Johns and Freshwater, 2005; Johns, 2000; Rolfe *et al.*, 2001; Todd and Freshwater, 1999; Van Ooijen, 2000). In addition some of the most widely used definitions of clinical supervision make reflective practice central to the aims of supervision. In 1994 Kohner, for example, identified the main purpose of clinical supervision as that of facilitating reflective practice within a patient-centered focus – a view that is supported by several authors who proposes that clinical supervision offers an ideal setting for the guidance of reflective practice.

Whilst some nursing commentators have questioned whether or not reflective practice needs to be an integral part of clinical supervision (Fowler and Chevannes, 1998), others have examined the relationship in detail. Todd and Freshwater (1999: 1383) for example examined the 'parallels and processes of a model of reflection in an individual clinical supervision session, and the use of guided discovery.' The authors advocate reflective practice as a model for clinical supervision 'because it provides safe space that facilitates a collaborative and empowering relationship which enables the practitioner to experience a journey of discovery in examining his/her everyday practice' (Todd and Freshwater, 1999: 1388). Heath and Freshwater (2000: 1298) used 'Johns' (1996) intent–emphasis axis to explore how a technical interest, misunderstanding of expert practice, and confusion of self awareness with counselling, can detract from the supervisory process.' They examined the nature of clinical supervision and reflective practice and how the two can combine effectively, especially when supervisors are reflective about their roles, and the clinical supervision experience is a guided reflection that enables deeper insights for the supervisee and supervisor.

On a slightly different track, Gilbert (2001: 199) focussed on the 'meticulous rituals of the confessional' and the potential for reflective practice and clinical supervision to act as 'modes of surveillance disciplining the action of professionals.' Using Foucault's (1982) concept of governmentality, Gilbert argued that, like governments, health settings act as 'forms of moral regulation' in which professionals exercise power through 'the complex web of discourses and social practices that characterize their work' (Gilbert, 2001: 199). In critiquing the discourses of empowerment (Gilbert, 2001: 205) that underlie the emancipatory intent of reflective practice and clinical supervision, he identifies the tendency of empowerment discourses to assume 'the existence of a damaged subject, traditional and rule bound [who] requires remedial work . . . to achieve forms of subjectivity consistent with modern forms of rule.'

Clouder and Sellars (2004: 262), writing from the perspective of physical therapists, used research conducted with undergraduate occupational therapy and physical therapy students to 'contribute to the debate about the functions of clinical supervision and reflective practice in nursing and other health care professions.' The authors responded to Gilbert's (2001) criticism of the sterility of debates about reflection and clinical supervision, and the potential for moral regulation and surveillance. They concluded that although both strategies make individuals more visible within the gaze of the workplace, Gilbert 'overlooked the possibility of resistance and the scope for personal agency within systems of surveillance that create tensions between personal and professional accountability.'

Freshwater (2005) to some extent agrees with Gilbert, in that she states: 'it could be posited that reflection guided through clinical supervision monitors the level of deviance from protocols, codes of conduct and policies, this through a confessional practice.' However, turning Foucault's theory back on itself she, like Clouder and Sellars (2004), points toward the scope for subversion and agency within the supervisory arrangement, providing examples of studies conducted in secure environments (Freshwater, 2005; Freshwater *et al.*, 2001, 2002).

It could be argued that this view is heavily dependent upon the orientation of the facilitator. Lahteenmaki (2005) observes that the supervision that students receive is closely related to their supervisor's view of the goals of learning; other writers concur with this view (see, for example, Van Ooijen, 2000). For example in the apprentice–master approach to learning, which relies heavily on the technical instrumental philosophy of education, the supervisee/practitioner is viewed as a passive recipient of knowledge. By way of contrast, reflective and critical approaches to learning, which emphasize the role of the supervisee/practitioner in analyzing and understanding their own practices, concentrate on eliciting the supervisee's espoused theories and values. To this end, reflective practice is an integral part of clinical supervision that focusses on facilitating learning through empowerment and emancipation (Freshwater, 2000; Taylor, 2002, 2004). Naturally, some individuals respond better to the apprentice–master approach to learning, finding reflection threatening and challenging, most often because it forces them to reflect on and develop an inner authority through the constant testing out of personal and relational hypotheses. But to argue for a supervision practice that either includes or dismisses reflective practice serves only to dichotomize the two concepts, and does little to acknowledge the interdependence of the two. Most experienced facilitators of learning would point out that the real skill of supervision in is integrating facilitative and directive skills to enable an optimal learning environment to suit the individual needs of the practitioner/learner.

Summary

In the earlier part of this chapter we referred to the personal nature of the reflective cycle and its importance in developing awareness and possibly stimulating the individual to adapt their behavior, if appropriate. We also discussed the concept of clinical supervision as a method of improving practice, and/or ensuring best practice, but also its potential to be used as a means of control and surveillance. We have looked at how the relationship between reflection and clinical supervision results in reflective practice and later added coaching as another form of reflection as a means of developing a reflective practitioner.

But, based on the input from those participating in the clinical supervision program referred to, and our experience over the years, there are many lessons to learn and questions to ask. *Clinical supervision should be work-related and aimed at improving practice and developing the individual. Supervision's focus should be practice-based,* allowing for exploration of the personal domain but always returning to the work-related topic, incorporating any new insights. Supervisees do not want to get bogged down in theoretical discussions: any models or theoretical frameworks are not intended to be prescriptive, but to provide support and clarity in what can sometimes be diffuse and complicated discussions.

Finally, whatever the underlying philosophical reasoning to introduce clinical supervision in a department, it is imperative that all parties are aware of the rules of play and commit to open and truthful communication.

References

ALG (Action Learning Group, West Midlands) (2006) Personal communication. See Walsh, E., Dilworth, S. and Freshwater, D. *Establishing Clinical Supervision in Prison Health Care Settings: Phase Three.* Bournemouth: Bournemouth University.

Benner, P. (1984) *From Novice to Expert. Excellence and Power in Clinical Nursing Practice.* Addison-Wesley, Menlo Park, CA.

Bishop, V. (2006) Clinical supervision: What is it? Why do we need it? in: Bishop, V. (ed.) *Clinical Supervision,* 2nd edn. Palgrave, Basingstoke.

Boeree, C.G. (2006) Personality theories: Abraham Maslow. *Psychology Department: Shippensberg University.* http://www.social-psychology.de/do/pt_maslow.pdf (11 January 2007).

Bond, M. and Holland, S. (1998) *Skills of Clinical Supervision for Nurses.* Open University Press, Buckingham, UK.

Boud, D., Cohen, R. and Walker, D. (2000) Introduction: Understanding learning from experience, in Boud, D., Cohen, R. and Walker, D. (eds) *Using Experience for Learning.* Open University Press, Buckingham, UK.

Burton, A.J. (2000) Reflection: nursing's practice and education panacea? *Journal of Advanced Nursing,* 31(5), 1009–17.

Carper, B.A. (1978) Fundamental patterns of knowing in nursing. *Advances in Nursing Science,* 1, 13–23.

Clouder, L. and Sellars, J. (2004) Reflective practice and clinical supervision: an interprofessional perspective. *Journal of Advanced Nursing,* 46(3), 262–9.

Cox, H., Hickson, P. and Taylor, B. (1991) Exploring reflection: knowing and constructing practice, in Gray, G. and Pratt, R. (eds) *Towards a Discipline of Nursing.* Churchill Livingstone, Melbourne.

Department of Health (1993) *A Vision for the Future. The Nursing, Midwifery and Health Visiting Contribution to Health and Health Care.* HMSO, London.

Driscoll, J. (2000) *Practising Clinical Supervision.* Baillière Tindall, London.

Espeland, K. and Shanta, L. (2001) Empowering versus enabling in academia. *Journal of Nursing Education,* 40(8), 342–6.

Fish, D. and Twinn, S. (1997) *Quality Clinical Supervision in the Health Care Professions.* Butterworth-Heinemann, Oxford.

Foucault, M. (1982) Afterword: the subject and power, in Dreyfus, H.L. and Robinow, P. (eds) *Beyond Structuralism and Hermeneutics.* Harvester Wheatsheaf, London.

Fowler, J. and Chevannes, M. (1998) Evaluating the efficacy of reflective practice within the context of clinical supervision. *Journal of Advanced Nursing,* 27(4), 379–82.

Freshwater, D. (2000) Transformatory Learning in Nurse Education. PhD thesis: University of Nottingham, Nottingham, UK.

Freshwater, D. (2005) Clinical supervision in the context of custodial care, in Freshwater, D. and Johns, C. (eds) *Transforming Nursing through Reflective Practice,* 2nd edn. Blackwell Publishing, Oxford.

Freshwater, D. (2007) Reflective practice and clinical supervision: two sides of the same coin? in Bishop, V. (ed.) *Clinical Supervision,* 2nd edn. Palgrave, Basingstoke, UK.

Freshwater, D., Walsh, L. and Storey, L. (2001) Developing leadership through clinical supervision in prison healthcare. *Nursing Management,* 8(8), 10.

Freshwater, D., Walsh, L. and Storey, L. (2002) Developing leadership through clinical supervision in prison healthcare. *Nursing Management*, 2, 10.

Gilbert, T. (2001) Reflective practice and clinical supervision: meticulous rituals of the confessional. *Journal of Advanced Nursing*, 36(2), 199–205.

Haber, J., Krainovich-Miller, B., McMahon, A. and Price-Hoskins, P. (1997) Cited in Espeland, K. and Shanta, L. (2001) Empowering versus enabling in academia. *Journal of Nursing Education*, 40(8), 342–6.

Hawkins, P. and Shohet, R. (1989) *Supervision in the Helping Professions: An Individual, Group and Organisational Approach*. Milton Keynes: Open University Press.

Heath, H. and Freshwater, D. (2000) Clinical supervision as an emancipatory process: avoiding inappropriate intent. *Journal of Advanced Nursing*, 32(5), 1298–306.

Holloway, E. (1995) *Clinical Supervision: A Systems Approach*. Sage, London.

Jarvis, P., Holford, J. and Griffin, C. (2001) *The Theory and Practice of Learning*. Kogan Paul, London.

Johns, C. (1996) Visualising and realising caring in practice through guided reflection. *Journal of Advanced Nursing*, 24(6), 1135–43.

Johns, C. (2000) *Becoming a Reflective Practitioner*. Blackwell Science, Oxford.

Johns, C. (2001) Depending on the intent and emphasis of the supervisor, clinical supervision can be a different experience. *Journal of Nursing Management*, 9(3), 139–45.

Johns, C. (2006) *Engaging Reflection in Practice: A Narrative Approach*. Blackwell Publishing, Oxford.

Johns, C. and Freshwater, D. (1998) *Transforming Nursing Through Reflective Practice*, 1st edn. Blackwell Science, Oxford.

Johns, C. and Freshwater, D. (2005) *Transforming Nursing Through Reflective Practice*, 2nd edn. Blackwell Science, Oxford.

Knowles, M.S. (1980) *The Modern Practice of Adult Education: From Pedagogy to Andragogy*. Prentice-Hall, Engelwood Cliffs, NJ.

Kohner, N. (1994) *Clinical Supervision in Practice*. Kings Fund Centre, London.

Lahteenmaki, M.L. (2005) Reflectivity in supervised practice: conventional and transformative approaches to physiotherapy. *Learning in Health and Social Care*, 4(1), 18–28.

Northcott, N. (2000) Clinical supervision – professional development or management control? in Spouse, J. and Redfern, L. (eds) *Successful Supervision in Health Care Practice*. Blackwell Science, Oxford.

NMC (Nursing and Midwifery Council) (2002) *Supporting Nurses and Midwives through Lifelong Learning*. Nursing and Midwifery Council, London.

Pesut, D.J. and Herman, J. (1999) *Clinical Reasoning: The Art and Science of Critical and Creative Thinking*. Delmar Publishers, New York.

Proctor, B. (1986) Supervision: a co-operative exercise in accountability, in Marken, M. and Payne, M. (eds) *Enabling and Ensuring – Supervision in Practice.* National Youth Bureau, Council for Education and Training in Youth and Community Work, Leicester, UK.

Rolfe, G., Freshwater, D. and Jasper, M. (2001) *Critical Reflection for Nursing and the Helping Professions: A User's Guide.* Palgrave, Basingstoke, UK.

Scheweer, E. (2000) *Veelzijdig coachen: Een praktische handleiding voor leidinggevenden en begeleiders.* Scriptum, Schiedam.

Schön, D.A. (1987) *Educating the Reflective Practitioner.* Jossey-Bass, San Francisco.

Spouse, J. and Redfern, L. (2000) Creating a quality service, in Spouse, J. and Redfern, L. (eds) *Successful Supervision in Health Care.* Blackwell Science, Oxford.

Taylor, B.J. (2000) *Reflective Practice: A Guide for Nurses and Midwives.* Open University Press, Maidenhead, UK.

Taylor, B.J. (2002) *Reflective Practice: A Guide for Nurses and Midwives,* 2nd edn. Open University Press, Maidenhead, UK.

Taylor, B.J. (2004) *Reflective Practice: A Guide for Nurses and Midwives,* 3rd edn. Open University Press, Maidenhead, UK.

Todd, G. and Freshwater, D. (1999) Reflective practice and guided discovery: clinical supervision. *British Journal of Nursing,* 8(20), 1383–98.

Van Ooijen, E. (2000) *Clinical Supervision: A Practical Guide.* Churchill Livingstone, Edinburgh.

Van Ooijen, E. (2003) *Clinical Supervision Made Easy.* Churchill Livingstone, Edinburgh.

Chapter 7

Reflective practice: the route to nursing leadership

Gwen Sherwood and Sara Horton-Deutsch

Introduction

Recommendations from *The Scholarship of Reflective Practice* resource paper (Taylor *et al.*, 2005) call for reflective models, theories and processes to develop transformative leaders. Leadership is the key ingredient in fostering healthy, nurturing environments. Creating a context for renewal and learning through reflection contributes to personal development and engagement in work that results in practice improvements and influences nurse satisfaction and retention. The dynamic contexts that define nursing and healthcare require transformational leaders who can modify the environment as both stabilizer and change agent. Incorporating reflection as a personal growth strategy expands emotional intelligence, an essential skill in transformative leadership. This chapter describes how critical reflection can help expand leadership capacity through personal development that leads to transformation.

Transformative leadership: a journey of the self

The view of leadership as an inner journey of the self is central to transformative leadership. Traditional descriptions of leadership have focussed on transactional activities such as managing people, processes and outcomes, all part of a supervisory role. In contrast, transformational leadership reframes the orientation to one of using the self in the leadership process of facilitating, coaching, mentoring and working with people to accomplish change in a value-based model. Transformational leaders engage in constant critical dialog to compare what they learn from experience matched against theoretical or ideal expectations, in essence, as critically reflective leaders (Sherwood and Freshwater, 2005).

Emergent leaders are in the forefront of change, able to create and influence dynamic, adaptive systems towards healthy work environments (Sherwood, 2003). Through reflection, practice leaders are able to match philosophy with action, overall mission with reality, and behaviors with consequences. Leadership is reflected in the environment created. The influences of transformational leadership become transparent in four elemental processes to discover meaning, create context, critically reflect on situations, and willfully engage in seeking one's 'internal compass' (Freshwater, 2004). The skills developed through emotional intelligence become the building blocks in the reflective, inner journey towards transformation as a critically reflective leader.

Discovering meaning

Transformative leaders develop emotional intelligence as part of the journey to find the true self (Vitello-Cicciu, 2002). Emotional intelligence emerges from a reflective process of self-discovery, self-awareness, self-management, motivation to contribute to something larger than oneself, and empathy for others' situation (Freshwater, 2004). Self-discovery moves into self-awareness and transcendence to be able to look outside one's own realm to respond to and help others. Meaning comes from the commitment to a cause greater than the self (see Chapter 9). Growth comes from reflectively monitoring one's responses to others and to situations with an expanding capacity for emotional intelligence. Transformative leaders concentrate on knowing the person and their individual development rather than exercising power over others. This unfolds in a reciprocal process of giving of oneself so as to inspire others to likewise give of themselves (Bolman and Deal, 2001). The very reciprocity inspires meaning and satisfaction.

Transformative leaders work from a sense of meaning, that is, from their inward spirit. The human spirit is one's inner essence, the defiant power that motivates and inspires questions of purpose, of how one experiences meaning, from engagement in one's work (Sherwood,

1997). Finding meaning requires a process of self-discovery to get a clear look at oneself, considering one's true potential, what one hopes for the future, and breaking long-held mental models. Reflections on and in actions are one pathway to self-discovery and transformation. Reflective questions ask: 'How do I typically respond to situations and events like this? What about this inspires me and gives me joy? What can I learn that will change my responses?'

Creating context

Work takes place in a given context, a work environment that influences how we respond to situations. Personal development is the core ingredient of the leadership journey, therefore, the workplace can only be transformed as the leader transforms his/her own self. Professional development through critical reflection offers a new approach for understanding individual differences, the work context and the organizational culture. Transformational leaders influence the workplace context and how care can be completed, and thus contribute to quality outcomes for patients as well as for workers.

In Chapter 2 we began to examine the nature of the relationship between culture and reflection. Culture is built from shared values and group behavior norms. Group behavior norms are the consequences of the usual ways group members interact and exist because of continued group reinforcement. Values influence decisions that shape what is considered normal for the group. All behaviors result in consequences. Group norms are reinforced by accepted consequences. To change behaviors, consequences have to change to reflect and reward the desired behaviors. The connection between behavior and consequences build the culture.

The economic focus in healthcare organizations has often created a culture that may be focussed on efficiency rather than on meaning from work, thus contributing to what Bolman and Deal (1997) term a loss of 'soul' that diminishes satisfaction. Reflection can help rebalance by asking tough questions about how mission is reflected in actions, philosophy matches priorities, behaviors connect with consequence, and the environment supports meaning from work.

Leaders must be able to create and manage the work environment as well as deconstruct the culture to change outcomes (Jones and Redman, 2000). A mismatch of personal values and organizational values lead to dissonance and dissatisfaction. When change is needed, reflection can unfreeze entrenched attitudes and behaviors. In seeking to reorder consequences of actions, one has to move beyond defending the present to a constructive analysis of the future, identify new ways of acting, and incorporate these strategies into a renewed culture.

Changing the culture means changing behaviors to match philosophy, mission and values with the realities of everyday work. Transformative leadership influences the interconnection of self, others, clients and systems by leading from a sense of mission with mindful presence so that it permeates the environment (Sherwood, 1997). It is developed through reflective practices that help to identify, clarify and promote individual strengths to maximize personal potential. Reflective leadership helps to create a transformative environment that is inviting, thus a 'place where people want to be.'

Reflecting about experience

There is no predetermined way to use reflection to discover and understand experience. Reflection is a personal journey of the self and is a critical aspect of the transformation journey to learn from one's actions, practice and way of being in a dynamic continuum of growth and development. Self-awareness is considered an essential aspect of effective reflection in which the self serves as the main instrument in the process. Reflection links cognitive behavioral skills in a cycle of self-monitoring, self-evaluating and self-reinforcing. Reflection fosters engagement with one's work. Reflection asks questions about the best response in situations. What is the right thing to do in this transaction? How can I best intervene in this situation? What does this person most need in this moment? What can I learn from this experience to help my response in the future? Leaders become aware of critical intent within a situation with the potential to change their usual response and thus bring the best self to practice.

Finding the internal compass: value-based leadership

Transformative leadership is value-based. Personal values are the foundation on which nurse leaders develop intrapersonal and interpersonal work with self and others. Philosophy is lived out in action; the stated mission matches reality; and behaviors are consistent with consequences. Value-based leadership is founded on respect for each individual. A reflective practice environment creates a space where participants can live their values and beliefs. Action theories that guide responses are modified from reflection on experience.

The inner compass directs value-based responses to circumstances and events. Acting consistently with one's values leads to inner strength and conviction, helping bridge gaps between the actual and ideal worlds. One constructs mental models or expectations of how something exists, thus creating one's own view of reality. Reflecting from a values-based orientation stimulates awareness of needed change. Change begins with awareness of one's mental model and the potential to recreate one's expectations and responses.

Living according to one's values contributes to meaning derived from one's work in the belief that one is contributing to something bigger than oneself. Leaders grounded in an inner core of spiritual meaning act from individual accountability combined with self-awareness that transcends mere cognitive responses and contributes to transformed environments. Reflective leaders see beyond the required techniques and skillful how-to of their work, reaching towards the deeper meaning and vision of the whole of their work experience. Reflective leaders constantly re-evaluate and re-establish their own internalized beliefs, values and norms. This is their way of defining and describing their own philosophical stance towards nursing work that results in performance improvement and leadership development. Leadership then begins with self-development, using reflective practice to locate the 'internal compass which guides leader actions, the inner core of being that guides and directs actions and practices' (Freshwater, 2004). The internal compass guides actions based on one's values and spirituality of meaning. It is through a reflective stance that the internal compass becomes the central voice of a person, thus the inspiration for consistently 'doing the right thing,' and defines professional artistry (Bolman and Deal, 1997).

The role of reflection in transformative leadership

Reflection is a generic term for the intellectual and affective activities through which individuals examine their experience to create and clarify meaning in terms of self, leading to a changed conceptual perspective. Reflective thinking is a rational and intuitive process which promotes positive change. Reflective thinking is an active process to carefully consider personal beliefs and present knowledge to recreate patterns for future actions. Leaders develop practical knowledge and working intelligence as they 'make sense' of their work when compared with known theoretical propositions. Reflection raises awareness to consider other, more effective ways to accomplish work, weighing evidence amid personal considerations. Reflection integrates self into one's work to expand leadership capacity.

Purpose of reflection

Reflection as a skill in nursing seeks to blend theory and practice. Professionals use reflection to uncover knowledge in and on action (Schön, 1983). In a spirit of inquiry one reflects on an experience to gain understanding of why and what happened so that future choices or actions will be handled more effectively. Reflection can help to make the most of multiple experiences by seeking meaning to inspire growth as one changes beliefs and expectations about future actions or perspectives.

In reflection, one has to let go of what one recalls about a critical incident in order to apply various cognitions to thinking, contemplating and analyzing to make sense of the experience (Taylor, 2000). Letting go can be a challenge in leadership, getting outside one's prevailing model or expectations to consider alternatives or other views. One seeks to make contextually appropriate changes by linking the cognitive behavioral skills of self-monitoring, self-evaluating and self-reinforcing. Critical thinking derives from a reflective stance to enable nurses to make sound decisions. It transcends 'doing' to emphasize 'being.'

Reflection becomes an integral part of continuous personal growth by helping nurses recognize and articulate learning (Davies, 1995). Reflection promotes cyclical rather than linear learning, asking questions about what one does, seeking new knowledge to answer questions, and integrating learning into leadership. Reflectively applying theory to practice helps fosters responsibility and accountability by changing responses to environmental cues (Wong *et al.*, 1997).

Reflecting to influence change

Self-awareness, self-monitoring, self-evaluating and self-reinforcing as described in emotional intelligence (Cherniss and Goleman, 2001) are critical skills for reflection (Kuiper and Pesut, 2004; Sherwood and Freshwater, 2005). Reflective thinking reviews an experience through a process of describing, analyzing and evaluating to inform actions in the future. Reflection can lead to changing one's mental models about practice which inform intentional, conscious and deliberative responses to environmental cues.

Just as learning is more than the content defining science and disease, practice is more than doing. Artistry in one's chosen work brings in multiple ways of acquiring knowledge. Carper (1978) identified the empirical, esthetic, personal and ethical ways of knowing as grounding the knowledge that informs nursing work. When applied to reflection, these four ways of knowing offer a structured way to think about how evidence clarifies work responses, accompanied by an awareness of how that work is accomplished (Burns and Bulman, 2000; Johns, 2004). Asking different questions from the various knowledge perspectives can reframe one's mental models about a phenomenon as a precursor to behavior change.

Professional development focuses on one's area of practice by critically examining real events in a comparison with ideal practice to re-engage from a new perspective (Teekman, 2000). The purposes of reflective practice can be integrated into any learning and development goal whether one's work is direct patient care provider, administrator or educator. Reflection can enable nurses to explore and come to understand the nature and boundaries of their own role and that of other health professionals (Freshwater, 2002; Johns, 1994, 1995).

Reflection to expand leadership capacity

Leadership and reflection have similar purposes. The primary aim of critical reflection and reflexivity are to create change and transformation, both of which are core functions of leadership. Both require presence and attentiveness to the moment, engagement in work, and willingness to be present. Both have a similar goal of creating positive work environments that enable all to thrive. Whereas traditional leadership methods seek to manage people and provide how-to strategies, transformative leadership is emergent with continuous cycles of reflective self-development.

Relationships are a critical part of nursing and positive relationships are part of a healthy environment that attracts workers. A transactional style of leadership, compared to a transformational approach, is linked to higher attrition (Thyer, 2003). Other studies also link reflective practice with developing clinical leadership skills and conclude that reflection should be a crucial element of any leadership and management program (Freshwater, 2002; Freshwater *et al.*, 2001).

Reflectively, leaders clarify their role and responsibilities within the situational context to determine whether they are on the right track. Thus, learning from experience contributes to 'know-how' or practical leadership knowledge. It moves one away from only relying on rule-based thinking that is self-limiting, and expands capacity towards expert leadership. The ability to move between theory and practice, selecting and transforming knowledge appropriate to the situation, is a mark of expertise, and illustrates a maturing practice in knowing how to use inquiry (Benner, 1984).

Principles of transformation

Twenty-first-century leadership demands are consistent with the process of individual transformation that comes from reflection. Cranton (1996) defined transformation as having three stages: self-directed learning, critical reflection and transformative learning. Self-directed learning sets the foundation for transformation as the learner takes responsibility and accountability for learning, moving forward through critical reflection to learn from experience by recalling, reflecting, analyzing, theorizing and recontextualizing to arrive at new conclusions and behaviors from a new understanding. Lastly, transformative learning comes from application. Here, through critical self-reflection in the inward journey of self-discovery, the learner articulates assumptions and questions those assumptions to move into meaningful perspectives.

Applied to leadership, the transformational process takes the learner into the inward journey of self-awareness. The journey of leadership is defined as a journey of self-development; no leader is stronger than his/her inner core of being. Leading the dynamics of change demands critically reflective leaders who are willing to engage in a constant critical dialog about their work. As such, transformational leadership contributes to healthcare improvement, what Graham (2003) describes as the cornerstone of clinical leadership.

Transformational leadership

Transformational leadership captures the elusive quality of leadership in which inner strength and character are cultivated by critically reflecting on challenging experiences. Developing a reflective stance for growth is an ongoing process of examining and questioning assumptions, values and perspectives and is an embedded skill for the transformational leader (Porter-O'Grady and Malloch, 2003). Transformational leaders must themselves understand the basics of change as well as lead others into the change process, thus transform situations by recognizing possibilities and designing new approaches, methods, or ways to think or act. Transformation results as new response patterns are embraced and become part of the routine. Transformative leaders have relational responsibilities to facilitate, coach and mentor others in their development. Relationship skills develop collaboration and communication with others to be able to influence, manage conflict, and build consensus and support (Barnsteiner *et al.*, 2007).

Reflection can help develop positive working relationships to build teamwork and collaboration, important contributors to healthcare quality (Cronenwett *et al.*, 2007). Leaders have a continual challenge to present with openness to diverse viewpoints and new approaches. Reflecting on experiences with others builds the skills of relational leadership to enable leaders to reach across disciplines and bring the work team together (Sherwood *et al.*, 2002). Self-awareness developed through a reflective stance builds relational skills that transform leaders through new views of:

- self gained through self-discovery;
- others as a community connected by dialog and communication;
- power that balances with influence and integrates value-based decision making; and
- the whole through a new understanding of values, mission and vision (Parker and Gadbois, 2000).

Reflective pause

How can reflection influence interactions with others?

How can you contribute to a nurturing work environment that encourages reflection and renewal?

Reflective models that impact leadership development

There is no one prescription for the reflective process. Reflection is a process of inquiry that involves a series of deeply regarded questions that can be processed before experience, during the experience, or after the event. For any method, the first stage is the awareness of the need for changing one's response and actions in a given circumstance. Reflection helps shape one's professional identify in relation to oneself, rather than being shaped by the environment. Leaders can use a questioning approach to address potential problems, thereby apprehending circumstances to control and monitor.

Self-questioning is a vital aspect of reflective thinking which helps clarify and categorize situations in order to begin to think logically in a particular circumstance and begin to uncover meaning from the encounter (Teekman, 2000). Using a structured process in reflective thinking lessens the possibility of overlooking important details. Reflection asks probing questions that stimulate reflection to elicit thinking, feelings, behaviors and doing (Burrows, 1995; Johns, 2000). Reflection is a personal process but may be most effective used in dialog with a coach, mentor or clinical supervisor who can help guide the discussion of events and help clarify values and beliefs and the effects on personal and professional practice (Wong *et al.*, 1997).

Three types of reflection

Taylor (2004) offers three types of reflection that are important to leadership development: technical, practical and emancipatory ways of reflecting. These can be used separately, or in any combination, according to the requirements of the practice or personal situation. Technical reflection acknowledges the influence of the scientific model in using empirical knowledge in daily nursing practice, improving clinical policies and procedures by devising reasoned approaches to work, and using critical thinking processes. Practical reflection offers a means of making sense of human interaction, offering the potential for change based on nurses' raised awareness of the nature of a wide range of communicative matters pertaining to their practice. Emancipatory reflection provides a systematic means of critiquing the status quo in the power relationships in the workplace, and it offers nurses raised awareness and a new sense of informed consciousness to bring about positive social and political change.

Reflection-on and in-action

Reflection-on-action is akin to mindfulness where one opens oneself to the moment by clearing out unwanted distractions and eliciting presence and openness before interacting with others. Reflection-on-action uses a retrospective stance to recall an event, to analyze and interpret the event, and to bring a knowledge base to examine the events. Freshwater (2002) cites the stages of becoming aware of uncomfortable thoughts and feelings, critically analyzing feelings against knowledge, giving rise to a new perspective. Reflection-in-action requires nurses to be conscious of what they are doing and how they are doing in that moment of practice (Horton-Deutsch, 2008, in press). It is complex with the need for self-monitoring to think before speaking and acting. It requires mindful presence in the moment of action. Processes for reflecting-in-action are those creative strategies that can be used at the time of interaction simultaneous with 'being, thinking, and doing.'

There are specific ways to develop skills to be reflective in the action moment. Examples include mindfulness, meditation or concentration in which one purposefully attends to the moment-to-moment experience. Through focussed attention one seeks calm and clarity of mind in leadership moments. This increases the capacity for integrating thoughts, facts and information in a way that reveals deeper, more integral wisdom. It is being able to stop for a moment to bring the self to bear in how to respond, knowing one's greater goal and purpose.

Three-stage model of reflection

The three-stage model of reflection can be easily applied to leadership development. The three stages use questions for progressively deeper analysis of the event: description of uncomfortable feelings and thoughts about a situation; critical analysis of feelings coupled with knowledge available; and reforming for a new perspective (Freshwater, 2002).

First, one describes the experience objectively, asking such questions as where it took place, who was there, when it occurred, what was said, what each participant did, and why each was present. Next, one analyzes the experience consistent with one's goals for personal growth, civic engagement and professional knowledge application. Questions include how one felt, assumptions made, expectations, past experiences, personal skills to draw upon. Finally, one articulates the learning that results to help change responses and actions in future situations.

Box 7.1 illustrates the series of questions that lead one through a critical reflection in the three-step model of reflection. Skills that enable one to take a reflective stance include self-awareness, ability to describe a situation, critical analysis, synthesis and evaluation.

Box 7.1 Three-step model of reflection.

1 Describe experience objectively
    Prompting questions may include:
    Where was I?
    Who else was there?
    When did the experience take place?
    What was said?
    What did I/others do?
    Why were we there?
2 Analyze experience in accordance with learning goals
    a Personal growth
        i   How did the experience make me feel?
        ii   What assumptions or expectations did I bring to the situation?
        iii How have past experiences influenced the manner in which I acted or responded?
        iv   Why did I/did I not experience difficulty working with others?
        v   What people skills do I draw on to handle situations? What skills would I like to have?
    b Civic engagement
        i   What was I/someone else trying to accomplish?
        ii   Did I/others act unilaterally or collaboratively, and why?
        iii What roles did each person in the situation play, and why?
        iv   How might someone else have interpreted the situation?
        v   How else could I have handled the situation?
        vi   What is the interest of the common good?
    c Professional knowledge
        i   What specific resources relate to the experience?
        ii   What similarities and differences are there between the perspective on the situation offered by the resources and the situation as it unfolded?
        iii How does this experience enhance my knowledge of specific reading, theory or concept?
3 Articulate learning
    a What did I learn?
    b How specifically did I learn it?
    c Why does this meaning matter?
    d How will I use this learning? What goals for self-improvement will I set as a result of this learning? How will it change my future experiences?

Applying leadership in action: reflection, integration and transformation

Reflection is an effective growth strategy for leaders who want to make a difference in the world around them. Transformative leaders bring together the spirit of inquiry that frames the reflective process with the awareness of the need for transforming actions and responses. The integration of personal growth with the enlightened action theories that guide how one enacts one's work gives way to transformation both personally and reflected in the culture. The focus of reflection is on personal growth through expanded emotional intelligence which considers oneself in community with others and lives with a greater purpose in mind. Strategies for self-management are the core of effective leadership. To experience transformation one has to experience change personally; for transformational leadership, one must first be transformed. Who we are is who we bring to work, and this self drives leadership capacity.

Reflective exercise

What are issues in nursing leadership and management that could benefit from reflective processes? Describe reflective processes and strategies for exploring these issues. Use the process and strategy selected to reflect on a practice story relating to a nursing leadership and management issue in which you were actively involved.

Reflection to develop leadership

To gain clarity about oneself requires focussed attention to foster greater calm and clarity of mind, increasing one's capacity for integrating thoughts, facts and information to evoke deeper, more integral wisdom. Reflection is a mirror to consider theory and ideal practice. It is a window to view and focus the self in the context of lived experience. It is a way to confront, understand and work toward resolution of desired practice and the reality. Reflecting on didactic and experiential learning helps bring together the juncture of theory and practice.

Integration into the culture

Recognizing, understanding and challenging the ways in which the historical, social, political and ethical context of professional practice is informed by and informs clinical decision-making processes facilitates the development of a leader who models a leader/researcher-based approach to improving and developing practice (Freshwater and Rolfe, 2001). Reflection is a problem-solving, intuitive process using interaction and a developmental process leading to transformation to see new views of oneself as well as those they influence. Transformative leaders work from a framework of internalizing, asking questions about what is happening, to be able to take on new views and organize new ways of doing things incorporating a global perspective.

Transformation for a new world view

Transformation creates a new way of thinking to uncover a new view of the world. Transformative leaders are capable of knowing and affirming those in shared disciplines, respecting diversity as well as common values, appreciating varied cultures and sharing common mission. Together they learn cooperatively from the experience of working together, listening, communicating effectively and embracing diversity in a growth-producing culture.

Leaders must engage in the processes of their work, not just absorb content and expert skills. Transformation is changing of world view, taking on new ways of collecting information, synthesizing and recontextualizing to find new meaning. It is taking accountability for one's learning. Meaning derives from reflection on creative work in which one must confront fears, break old patterns and seek self-discovery. It requires reflective evaluation of oneself, looking at one's potential, preferred direction, repressed hopes, and fantasies of the future.

The role of the nurse leader in the healthcare arena is to create context for the work of nursing. Leaders work together in achieving mission at all levels of the organization, regardless of the setting. Purpose-driven workers encounter new situations with new potentials by honoring values and mission. Healthcare constantly balances competing values and demands while honoring mission and ensuring survival, making tough decisions amid tight resources. Transformational leadership, with leaders who create lasting change, begins as a journey of the self (Bolman and Deal, 2001).

Summary

Improvements and progress often only come about following unsettling circumstances that challenge our status quo (Ross *et al.*, 2005).

We all act in the context of particular circumstances and past experiences and reflect on events afterwards, reacting according to a set pattern. Work environments are dynamic, never static, and open to ever shifting contexts. Reflection is a primary method for dealing with the constancy of change that leaders face daily (Porter-O'Grady, 1992). By viewing change as a constant, one can maintain a reflective stance in which change is valued and embraced. Healthcare requires knowledge workers who recognize the generativity of transformative leadership, coaching, facilitating, and developing self and others.

Reflection requires time, effort and ongoing commitment if one is to gain deeper insights to make lasting changes in one's work. Transformational leadership helps in creating an environment that facilitates caring and thoughtful interactions with others as instruments in positive practice outcomes. It leads to an environment that encourages openness, flexibility and efficiency to achieve outcome goals of professional renewal, satisfaction and retention.

In summary, leadership that guides an organization through turbulent times must be able to break out of the box to see a new version of the present reality, thus viewing the workplace and its workers with a new lens. Transformational leaders create the possibility of building a culture that promotes the autonomy, communication and recognition that fosters a satisfied workforce.

References

Barnsteiner, J., Disch, J., Hall, L., Mayer, D. and Moore, S. (2007) Promoting interprofessional education. *Nursing Outlook*, 55(3), 144–50.

Benner, P. (1984) *From Novice to Expert: Uncovering the Knowledge Embedded in Clinical Practice*. Addison-Wesley, Boston, MA.

Bolman, L.G. and Deal, T.E. (1997) *Reframing Organizations: Artistry, Choice, and Leadership*, 2nd edn. Jossey-Bass, San Francisco.

Bolman, L.G. and Deal, T.E. (2001) *Leading with Soul*. Jossey-Bass, San Francisco.

Burns, S. and Bulman, C. (2000) *Reflective Practice in Nursing: The Growth of the Professional Practitioner*, 2nd edn. Blackwell Science, London.

Burrows, D. (1995) The nurse teacher's role in the promotion of reflective practice. *Nurse Education Today*, 15, 346–50.

Carper, B.A. (1978) Fundamental patterns of knowing in nursing. *Advances in Nursing Science*, 1(1), 13–23.

Cherniss, C. and Goleman, D. (eds) (2001) *The Emotionally Intelligent Workplace: How to select for, measure, and improve emotional intelligence in individuals, groups, and organizations*. Jossey-Bass, San Francisco.

Cranton, P. (1996) *Professional Development as Transformative Learning: New Perspectives for Teachers of Adults.* Jossey-Bass, San Francisco.

Cronenwett, L., Sherwood, G., Barnsteiner, J., Disch, J., Johnson, J., Mitchell, P., Sullivan, D.T. and Warren, J. (2007) Quality and safety education for nurses. *Nursing Outlook*, 55(3), 122–31.

Davies, E. (1995) Reflective practice: a focus for caring. *Journal of Nursing Education*, 34(4), 167–74.

Freshwater, D. (ed.) (2002) *Therapeutic Nursing: Improving Patient Care Through Reflection.* Sage, London.

Freshwater, D. (2004) Reflection: a tool for developing clinical leadership. *Reflections on Nursing Leadership*, 2nd quarter, 20–6.

Freshwater, D. and Rolfe, G. (2001) Critical reflexivity: a politically and ethically engaged method for nursing. *NT Research*, 6(1), 526–37.

Freshwater, D., Walsh, L. and Storey, L. (2001) Developing leadership through clinical supervision in prison healthcare. *Nursing Management*, 8(8), 10.

Graham, I. (2003) Leading the development of nursing within a Nursing Development Unit: the perspectives of leadership by the team leader and a professor of nursing. *International Journal of Nursing Practice*, 9(4), 213–22.

Horton-Deutsch (2008) Thinking it through: the path to reflective leadership. *American Nurse Today* (accepted for publication).

Johns, C. (1994) Nuances of reflection. *Journal of Clinical Nursing*, 3, 71–5.

Johns, C. (1995) Framing learning through reflection within Carper's fundamental ways of knowing in nursing. *Journal of Advanced Nursing*, 22, 226–34.

Johns, C. (2000) *Becoming a Reflective Practitioner.* Blackwell Science, Oxford.

Johns, C. (2004) Becoming a transformational leader through reflection. *Reflections on Nursing Leadership*, 2nd quarter, 24–6.

Jones, K. and Redman, R. (2000) Organizational culture and work redesign: experiences in three organizations. *Journal of Nursing Administration*, 30(12), 604–10.

Kuiper, R. and Pesut, D. (2004) Promoting cognitive and metacognitive reflective reasoning skills in nursing practice: self-regulated learning theory. *Journal of Advanced Nursing*, 45(4), 381–91.

Parker, K. & Gadbois, S. (2000) Building community in the healthcare workplace. *Journal of Nursing Administration*, (9), 426–31.

Porter-O'Grady, T. (1992) Transformational leadership in an age of chaos. *Nursing Administration Quarterly*, 17(1), 17–24.

Porter-O'Grady, T. and Malloch, K. (2003) *Quantum Leadership: A Textbook of New Leadership.* Jones & Bartlett, Boston, MA.

Ross, A., King, N. and Firth, J. (2005) Interprofessional relationships and collaborative working: encouraging reflective practice. *Online Journal of Issues in Nursing*, 10(1), 4.

Schön, D. (1983) *The Reflective Practitioner: How Practitioners Think in Action.* Basic Books, New York.

Sherwood, G. (1997) Patterns of caring: the healing connection of interpersonal harmony. *International Journal for Human Caring*, 1(1), 30–8.

Sherwood, G. (2003) Leadership for a healthy work environment: caring for the human spirit. *Nurse Leader*, 1(5), 36–40.

Sherwood, G. and Freshwater, D. (2005) Doctoral education for transformational leadership in a global context, in Ketefian, S. and McKenna, H. (eds) *Doctoral Education in Nursing: International Perspectives*. Routledge, London.

Sherwood, G., Thomas, E., Simmons, D. and Lewis, P. (2002) A teamwork model to promote patient safety in critical care. *Critical Care Nursing Clinics of North America*, 14, 333–40.

Taylor, B. (2000) *Reflective Practice: A Guide for Nurses and Midwives*. Allen & Unwin, UK; Open University Press, Melbourne, Australia.

Taylor, B. (2004) Technical, practical and emancipatory reflection for practising holistically. *Journal of Holistic Nursing*, 22(1), 73–84.

Taylor, B., Freshwater, D., Horton-Deutsch, S. and Sherwood, G. (2005) *The Scholarship of Reflective Practice*. Sigma Theta Tau International Press. Position Paper (http://www.nursingsociety.org/about/resource_reflective.doc).

Teekman, B. (2000) Exploring reflective thinking in nursing practice. *Journal of Advanced Nursing*, 31(5), 1125–35.

Thyer, G. (2003) Dare to be different: transformational leadership may hold the key to reducing the nursing shortage. *Journal of Nursing Management*, 11(2), 73–9.

Vitello-Cicciu, J.M. (2002) Exploring emotional intelligence: Implications for nursing leaders. *Journal of Nursing Administration*, 32(4), 203–10.

Wong, F., Loke, A., Wong, M., Tse, H., Kan, E. and Kember, D. (1997) An action research study into the development of nurses as reflective practitioners. *Journal of Nursing Education*, 36, 476–81.

Part III

Using reflection to enhance teaching and learning

Chapter 8

Reflective practice and therapeutic use of self

Dawn Freshwater, Philip Esterhuizen and Sara Horton-Deutsch

Introduction

We have already written of the theory–practice gap in nursing, in relation to both educational and professional practices. The external polarization described between theory and practice has also been identified as reflective of an internal split, deeply embedded psychologically within the practitioner (Freshwater, 2000, 2002; Menzies-Lyth, 1970, 1988). Reflective practice, we have posited, is one way of bridging the theory–practice gap. In the context of this chapter this bridging could be seen as the outer manifestation of the inner repair that might also be taking place. It could be argued that the resistance or struggle to bring together theory and practice in nursing speaks not only to the lack of integration in education, research and practice, but also to the resistance of nurses themselves to become conscious of and live with the tensions or anxieties within their everyday practice and within themselves. In this chapter we develop the notion of the therapeutic self, relating this to the theory–practice gap, which we believe needs to be addressed not only from the outside in but also from the inside out and that this (lifetime) work is a fundamental driver and outcome of critical reflection.

Mind the gap

The work of Isobel Menzies-Lyth (1970) on psychological defenses in social systems highlighted an internal splitting process. Her work with doctors, nurses and administrators in hospital settings found that they viewed patients as objects in order to be able to cope with their strong and often ambivalent feelings towards them. The closer and more concentrated the relationship with the patient, the more likely the nurse was to experience anxiety. The process of splitting off feelings is both an inner and outer process (Briant and Freshwater, 1998). Thus the nurse manages her anxiety by splitting her feelings off both from herself (inner world) and from her patients (outer world) (Menzies-Lyth, 1970). As a result of this splitting off the nurse can become dis-identified with aspects of her own psyche and/or bodily experience. The nurse is therefore disconnected from the source of her caring – the self. This inner split was also found to be inherent in the nursing service, which advocated splitting up contact with the patient through task allocation. This was certainly our experience as early on in nursing we found ourselves carrying out the 'observations' whilst another nurse would approach the same patient to perform 'wound care.' The same patient would be greeted by yet another new face for their 'pressure area care.'

However we view this system of work now, it is important to place this – now old-fashioned – task-related method of nursing in a social and historical perspective. It is with some degree of hindsight that we can now interpret it as being alienating and dis-identifying, although this was not the initial philosophy at its introduction. Lee (1979) discusses how this form of nursing followed an industrial model clustering aspects of care into groups with responsibility based on skill and seniority. Interestingly, from the perspective of oppression, allocation of tasks was awarded status from within the profession based on the hierarchical structure mirroring the military origins of nursing (Dolan *et al.*, 1983).

While on the issue of task-centered care, an important argument supporting this system was that all aspects of care would be provided. However, Lelean's (1973) research indicated the contrary and highlights one of the weaknesses; namely that nursing staff worked to sign off their work books, rather than provide care for their patients. The point we are trying to make here is that task-centered nursing was less about consciously depersonalizing nursing staff and more about discipline and getting the job done to the best possible standard by the person best suited, in the quickest possible time. Within the historical and social context of the time, this was considered state-of-the-art, top-quality patient care. Interestingly it could be argued that nurses still resort to task-centered care when short-staffed as it is, apparently, seen as being the more efficient method of working (Esterhuizen, 1997).

Sadly, some of Menzies-Lyth's findings still hold strong today, with many nurses preferring 'busyness' and 'doing' to 'relating' and 'being.' It was only 20 years ago that Menzies-Lyth (1988) noted that, although some things had changed in the organization of nursing, there were no major changes. She continues to argue that nurses require legitimate opportunities to understand their personal feelings, perceptions and anxieties. For many British nurses a new era opened for them on reading Steven Wright's book, *My Patient – My Nurse* (1994). It provided them with the *permission* to think through what they wanted to achieve with their care and footholds on how to move away from task orientation. In America, Watson's seminal work *Nursing: Human Science and Human Care* (1988) provided similar insights – namely that as a nurse you were an active part of the equation, could not objectify the patient, and you were actually changed and altered due to your interaction with the patient.

In the same timeframe Jacobs (1988) further argued that the struggle to polarize object from subject involves denial and repression of self; this is energy sapping and takes up psychic space, leaving the individual practitioner with less of her emotional self available, either for herself or her patients or, perhaps as important, for the argument for the process of learning. This too, needs to be placed in context as, historically, nurses have been selected on the basis of their submissive and non-assertive character traits rather than their intellectual prowess, and these 'nursing characteristics' appear to have been propagated through to the present day (Birchenall, 2003; Kirby, 2003; Lorentzon, 2003; Wilson and Startup, 1991).

Feeding into this idea of nurses being submissive, in an exploratory study using the Friel Co-dependence Assessment Inventory and the modes of Roy's adaptation model, Chappelle and Sorrentino (1993) show that while 160 nurses show responsibility, 65 show varying degrees of co-dependent behavioral characteristics. Bennett *et al.* (1992) quote published co-dependency figures among nurses as ranging between 75% and 90%. They suggest that nursing serves, by virtue of its caring nature and its altruistic and ascetic origins, to attract those with a disposition to co-dependency (Hall and Wray, 1989; Malloy and Berkery, 1993; Sherman *et al.*, 1989; Yates and McDaniel, 1994). However, more recent literature questions these figures. Hopkins and Jackson (2002) and Martsolf (2002) suggest that this is not the case. Hopkins and Jackson (2002) found the incidence of co-dependent behavior among nursing students no higher than among their contemporaries on other courses – they were, however, researching students and their learning in the academic setting and not in the hospital setting. Biering's

(1998) findings, using a cohort of eight Registered Nurses, indicate that these nurses, coming from dysfunctional families, had developed skills which could be put to good use within the healthcare setting and the findings do not support the assertion that these nurses were co-dependent in their own behavior.

Whilst we may appear to be fairly critical in our exposition, we are also careful to care for professional colleagues for we do not wish to be part of the oppressing force we mention. Taylor *et al.* (1999) address important issues, namely the stress and decline in morale nurses experience at not being able to care for their patients and their frustration at not having the resources to adequately deal with patients' suffering due to reduced staffing levels. Although, as will be discussed in due course, nurses are often perceived as an oppressed and powerless group, reflecting on our own reasons for staying in the nursing profession, we are aware of a sense of belonging. More importantly, the perception of unconditional reciprocity seemed to instill (and fit with) a feeling of being and self which relates to work published by Nåden and Eriksson (2000, 2002, 2004), Spouse (2001), Stickley and Freshwater (2002) and Widdershoven (1999).

Being available

The ability to be available and create space for therapeutic work are fundamental to the implementation of reflective practice (Johns, 1998) and substantiate the dimensions discussed by Knowles (1980) (Table 8.1) which add up to a quest for self-actualization and tie in with the perception that learning is an individual and transformational process.

Several authors note that self-awareness is an essential component of the reflective process (Atkins and Murphy, 1993; Freshwater, 2000, 2002; Mezirow, 1981; Schön, 1983). The development of self-awareness however is something that requires structured time and space for self-reflection as indicated in Schön's model 2 learning (Schön, 1983). This is something that nurse education, despite its acknowledgment of reflective practice, does not easily provide, either in clinical practice or in educational institutions. Whilst the current argument for structured time for reflection in the form of clinical supervision is to some extent addressing this issue (Bishop, 2007; Bond and Holland, 1998; Freshwater, 2003, 2007; Johns, 1998; see Chapter 6), this process is beset with its own difficulties. If we are to believe that the findings of Menzies-Lyth (1970) still hold some credibility today, then could it be that nursing per se might find the space and time to reflect on self and

Table 8.1 Dimensions of maturation (Knowles, 1980: 29).

From	Toward
1 Dependence	Autonomy
2 Passivity	Activity
3 Subjectivity	Objectivity
4 Ignorance	Enlightenment
5 Small abilities	Large abilities
6 Few responsibilities	Many responsibilities
7 Narrow interests	Broad interests
8 Selfishness	Altruism
9 Self-rejection	Self-acceptance
10 Amorphous self-identity	Integrated self-identity
11 Focus on particulars	Focus on principles
12 Superficial concerns	Deep concerns
13 Imitation	Originality
14 Need for certainty	Tolerance for ambiguity
15 Impulsiveness	Rationality

therein practice an uncomfortable pastime? These and related concepts are central to the development of this study and their relevance to the process of nursing and nurse education have been expanded upon in Chapters 3 to 6.

Having a self

The literature on the topic of self is large and diverse. It ranges from theories of self in philosophical terms, to theories of self in psychological terms, to spiritual and transpersonal theories (Wilber, 1981) to biological theories. The concept of self which a person possesses is a product of both personal reflection and social interaction. Dawson (1998) cites Priest's (1991) definition of the self as:

> *an individual that is conscious of the individual that it is while at the same time being conscious that it is the individual it is conscious of.* (p. 163)

The self is an important concept in nursing as often when patients are ill, either physically or psychologically, the self-concept is challenged. According to Dawson (1998) the most striking and consistent feature reported is a changed self-concept. Dawson (1998) goes on to argue that the concept of self most commonly used in nursing is one of

Cartesian duality. These comments are harmonious with those of nursing theorists Parse (1987), Rogers (1970) and Newman (1994).

The experiencing self as described by Bohart (1993) and Maddi (1989) is essentially anti-reductionist in nature. Life is apprehended through experiencing, which involves an interplay of thought and feeling, without either of these concepts being conceived of as polar opposites (Bohart, 1993). Humanistic psychologists describe the self as conceived of separate entities. Rogers (1991) for example speaks of the organismic self and the self-concept. The organismic self is that aspect of the self which is essentially the real inner life of the person and is present from birth. The organismic self consists of the basic force which regulates the individual's physiological and psychological growth; growth and maturity are seen as the central aims of this aspect of the self (Hough, 1994; Rogers, 1991). Therefore the focus of the organismic self is essentially internal.

According to Burns (1982: 9) self-concept is 'forged out of the influences exerted on the individual from outside, particularly from people who are significant others.' This definition is in accord with the humanistic school of psychology, which views the self-concept as the individual's perception of himself, based on life experience and the way he sees himself reflected in the attitudes of others (Rogers, 1991). The self-concept is acquired very early in life and is continually reinforced by ongoing communications with significant others throughout life. As the self develops it needs to feel loved and accepted and as a result the organismic self is neglected in favor of the self-concept.

The bridging of the theory–practice gap could be seen as the outer manifestation of the inner repair that could also be taking place. Perhaps the resistance of the coming together of theory and practice in nursing speaks not only to the lack of integration in education and practice, but also to the resistance of nurses themselves to become conscious of and live with the tensions or anxieties within their everyday practice and within themselves. It is argued that the theory–practice gap needs to be addressed not only from the outside in but also from the inside out and it is this that will be developed as a theme in the course of this work.

Inner conflict

The concept of the theory–practice gap being a manifestation of the individual's inner conflict is one that needs to be looked at more closely. When confronted with the realities of work in the clinical setting, nursing students can lose touch with their personal values, and losing touch with their personal values can lead to alienation from themselves. Helkama *et al.* (2003) discuss a decline and changes in moral reasoning during the education of medical students, while Allcock and Standen (2001), Greenwood (1993) and MacIntosh (2003) discuss possible desensitization that student nurses undergo during their education which could have strong moral implications for the quality of care delivered. In the case of the participants in Esterhuizen's (2007) study who completed the program, although they adapted initially to ward cultures, they always seemed aware of the fact that they were adapting to something they did not agree with – they seemed almost to have a strategic approach to their development and the points at which they extended and/or set their boundaries (Esterhuizen, 2007).

With regard to self-actualization, students in the same research who completed the program seemed, from a point roughly midway, able to differentiate good care from bad and were aware when they were compromising themselves as individuals and professionals (Esterhuizen, 2007). They were able to deal with problems and challenges as they arose without personalizing them and in some cases it was quite clear that they were not prepared to invest energy in situations they thought were not worth the effort. By the end of the program the students had become autonomous and self-sufficient and all articulated a change in their level of communication with others. They were aware of their own boundaries, seemed unprepared to compromise their professional integrity and were self-confident and assertive to challenge. The above-mentioned characteristics, exhibited by the students at the end of the program, correlate with work by Maslow on self-actualization (Boeree, 2006). Knowles (1980), in his work on the dimensions of maturation (Table 8.1), discusses an individual's move from superficial to deep concerns, moving away from a focus on particulars towards a focus on principles and from impulsiveness to rationality. This parallels Maslow's idea of differentiating between good and bad from a professional perspective and being unprepared to compromise personal and professional integrity. The students' ability to deal with problems and challenges illustrates their ability to objectify situations and think more broadly, accepting ambiguity and making choices to invest in dialog they perceived was important. They had become more autonomous in their decision making and enlightened in their view of the world – in other words, they seemed to have integrated their self-identity and were more self-accepting of their abilities, strengths and weaknesses. In many ways this could be described as inside-out learning, learning from the inside out, or as previously discussed, deep learning (Greenwood, 1998), transformational learning (Freshwater, 2000) and emancipatory reflection (see Chapter 2).

Self-esteem

In order to feel empowered, the nurse first needs to become aware of or understand what it means to be disempowered, and also importantly of the ways that they may be disempowering themselves. This requires that the nurse knows themselves as subject, and thereby the patient as subject, implying that nursing practice is a subjective experience.

Johns (1998) has challenged the process of nurse education for its lack of attention to the social forces that serve to oppress nurses, claiming that this could be a projection of their own lack of voice. Could it be that nurse education is itself a form of oppression by the very fact that it does not attend to this issue? It is proposed here that nurse education should attend to this issue immediately; nurse teachers need to find their own voice in order to empower their students. One way nurse teachers can do this is by examining their own contradictions in educational practices and making their beliefs and values known through their work. When taking Knowles' (1980) 'dimensions of maturation' (Table 8.1) into account, it is clear that an educationalist in both academic and clinical areas has an important responsibility to build the student's self-esteem. Espeland and Shanta (2001) suggest that faculty staff confuse 'empowering' with 'enabling' and often provide too much support to students, resulting in a form of interdependency between student and staff. This initial relationship built between faculty and student in the academic setting can provide the student with a false sense of security and lead to a cultural shock when confronted by the realities of the clinical setting (Smith and Gray, 2001a; Spouse, 2001). The student needs to be prepared to deal with the demands and rigors of the nursing profession, to have the courage to operate a personal philosophy of care and to be able to liaise with colleagues in the ward setting without adapting thoughtlessly to the new situation or feeling victimized (Holland, 1999; Johns, 1995a; MacIntosh, 2003; Smith and Gray, 2001b; Stickley and Freshwater, 2002; Watson *et al.*, 1999).

Nurses in practice, like teachers, often live with contradictions regarding their desired practice and the practice that they can carry out in reality (Johns, 1995b). Although some autonomy is afforded the nurse practitioner, many decisions are still perceived as resting with the doctor. The locus of control is seen as external (Rotter, 1966, 1971). This impacts work performance, as Mullins (1989) clearly articulates in his discussion around the attribution theory of motivation. Nurses, however, do not remain completely silent within their practice; in the struggle to have their voice heard, a game is often played (Berne, 1991; Stein, 1967, 1978; Stein *et al.*, 1990). The 'game' goes something like this: the nurse make a suggestion to the doctor in such a way that the doctor seems to have made the suggestion themselves; if the doctor joins in, then all parties feel happy and the patient gets the care that the nurse believes to be appropriate. If the doctor opts out of the game, the nurse is left feeling frustrated and may still carry out the care that she believes to be appropriate, ignoring the doctor, or alternatively she will carry out the doctor's orders, ignoring herself. The nurse may then become angry with herself for 'giving in' or playing the game; at times she may take her anger out on the patient. The model of transactional analysis offers a useful perspective on this game; the nurse can shift between rebellious child and compliant child and nurturing parent and critical parent. The doctor also takes his share of roles on the stage (Berne, 1991; Hough, 1994). This is not to say that nursing practice is never based on adult decisions, nor that nurses always feel powerless. Indeed, choosing to play the game represents an active stance, whether the choice is conscious or unconscious.

The transpersonal relationship

Work by Nåden and Eriksson (2000, 2002, 2004) addresses the powerful position a nurse can assume in entering into a relationship with the patient in a way that showcases the art of her profession. The transpersonal relationship and the, often, unspoken communication between the nurse and her patient allow both parties to 'be' in the space that they fill. One 60-year-old patient shared the following insights during a dialog:

> *I wasn't just one more patient passing through this bed, but an equal whom she respected . . . It was apparent in her whole attitude – her humility for the patient. Gentle! Open! Close! I have thanked her for what she has been for me.* (Nåden and Eriksson, 2000: 25)

Nåden and Eriksson go on to suggest that, where the language of sensitivity exists, suffering is alleviated because the nurse has confirmed the patient and given her room to suffer. This is, to me, a prime example of therapeutic self – the nurse not attempting to take on the patient's suffering as her own, but understanding that it is 'sufficient' to be unconditionally present in the moment.

In Esterhuizen's (2007) research a similar situation arose. A student decided to accompany a foreign patient, with whom she could not communicate, to the chapel as she felt, based on the patient's history, that the patient had been severely traumatized and had seen her agitatedly playing with a rosary. As the student approached the chapel, they could see an almost life-size white marble statue of the Virgin Mary, at which point the patient began to clap and sing and cry – an outpouring of emotion. The student slowed before wheeling the patient into the main body of the chapel. Once inside, the patient again showed an emotional outpouring of (what appeared to be) grief and religious ecstasy. The student apparently did 'nothing,' she was 'just with the patient.' This resonates with the work by Watson (1988) and Nåden and Eriksson (2000, 2002) who speak of unconditionally 'being with.' The student in this situation had no notions of these writings, but was following her intuition and what felt right to her (Esterhuizen, 2007).

These vignettes illustrate that actively choosing is an intrinsic factor within human action whether preceded by reflection or not (Burns, 1982) – in these situations, the active choice to care for another person.

Although there are gems that illustrate the individual's maturity and self-actualization there is, unfortunately, a substantial amount of evidence to support the notion that nurses have been and continue to feel oppressed; whether or not this is real (external) or imaginary (internal) is open to debate, the fact remains that it impacts retention and recruitment and thereby continuity of care (Fisher *et al.*, 1994; Friedson, 1970; Roberts, 1983; Scott, 1998). Spencer (1986) observed that employees, when feeling oppressed, chose to leave and go to a competitor, which was viewed as relatively safe behavior. Alternatively, the employee could attempt to change the situation through direct action and voicing. This was felt to be more risky. Freshwater's (1998) research study, drawing upon critical theory, posits that reducing the theory–practice gap through reflective practice and self-awareness provides an opportunity to address the perceived power imbalance through voicing and action which in turn directly and indirectly affects practice. In support of Johns' (1998) work in which he criticizes nursing education's lack of attention to educating nurses to deal with the (political) rigors of practice, Espeland and Shanta (2001) aptly discuss the role and responsibility of the nurse educator with regard to empowering students and cite Glass (1998) as suggesting three necessary components:

> *. . . the raising of consciousness, the development of a strong positive esteem, and the political skills need [sic] to negotiate and change the health-care system.*

Some parties support the idea of the student being an agent to change the status quo in healthcare, but this requires the academic and ward staff to want to change practice themselves and 'use' the student as a change agent in the most positive way – the student is then a source of new (theoretical) ideas and of ideological inspiration. Unfortunately, this is not the case in many instances. Education tends to dictate rather than coach (Carlson-Catalano, 1992; Clare, 1993; Leyshon, 2002; Litchfield, 2001) and registered staff in practice settings appear threatened when confronted by change (Randle, 2003).

Freire (1972) introduced the world of education to the notion of conscientization. Freire (1972) presented conscientization as the ability to become critically conscious. This is not simply examining an event to see how it could have been done differently; critical consciousness is linked to critical awareness and implies a political dimension, which enables assumptions inherent in ideologies to be challenged. Freire (1972) suggests that 'false consciousness,' that is, consciousness that is culturally induced within individuals, can be transcended by education. This implies that there is a consciousness that is not culturally induced; this could be interpreted as referring to the authentic self, what Rogers (1991) refers to as the organismic self as opposed to the self-concept. However, we believe that even the organismic self is to some extent culturally influenced, perhaps through what Jung terms the collective unconscious (Jung, 1960).

The central tenet of Freire's pedagogy (1972) is the practice of transcending false consciousness in order to achieve conscientization, interpreted by Askew and Carnell (1998: 65) as 'coming to a consciousness of oppression and a commitment to end that oppression.' Mezirow (1975, 1981), when discussing adult education, refers to this as perspective transformation. However, becoming conscious of one's oppression and making the commitment to end it require two different shifts. We would argue (as did Menzies-Lyth 20 years ago) that there is an enormous resistance to coming to consciousness and ending uncritical acceptance through action.

Action does not always equate with taking responsibility for the self against the perceived oppressor (reclaiming power explicitly); it may in fact mean choosing to remain unconscious (powerless) or consciously playing the power game (playing with the implied power). The latter is particularly employed by students (at all levels).

Nurses, like other groups throughout history, have been described as an oppressed group (Roberts, 1983). The cultural narration of nurses is to be subordinate. This view is supported by a wealth of literature, which advocates that nurses lack autonomy and control (Friedson, 1970), lack self-esteem (Greenleaf, 1978), fear success (LeRoux, 1978) and subscribe to the submissive–aggressive syndrome (Stein, 1978). It could be argued that the infiltration of nursing theory with the mechanistic model of medicine previously highlighted is evidence to support this viewpoint. Johns (1995b) refers to this as the barrier of medical hegemony to nursing autonomy. (Hegemony refers to the extent to which there is uncritical acceptance of the dominant groups, meaning systems, within the healthcare culture; Grundy, 1987.) Roberts (1983) asserts that the education system is one of the mechanisms that reinforces this position stating that: 'if the education is controlled by the powerful and limited to the curricula that support their values, little conflict occurs' (p. 24). However, as above, it could be argued that students are only able to challenge the prevailing values from a position of consciousness that is of their own values.

Conflict does occur, although not necessarily overtly. The conflict manifests itself in other ways, often as internalized self-deprecation, resulting in low self-esteem. Individuals may not be aware that some internalized self-criticism originates in uncritical acceptance and unexpressed conflict in relation to feeling oppressed. Thus, a false consciousness develops, sometimes without the individual knowing that there may be a different consciousness. In addition to this, situations of horizontal violence (a topic that is being more openly discussed in nursing circles) may arise (Farrell, 1997; Freshwater, 2000).

The notion of a false consciousness derived from Hegel and Marx is not necessarily a helpful concept, for as Johns (1998a) discusses, the notion of a false consciousness implies that there is a true consciousness. Although this might be correct, it could be added that any shift in consciousness is relative and is never an end in itself; the notion of the self-concept may provide a more helpful term (Burns, 1982; Rogers, 1991). Perhaps the shift relates more to matching the inner and the outer worlds more closely, bringing the personal and professional theories more in relation, to achieve more congruent and authentic action. One might ask: what is it that facilitates this shift in consciousness? In the context of this book, we contend that reflective practice, or rather critical reflection, is one way of both raising and shifting consciousness.

Freire (1972) posited two phases to the process of liberation from oppression: first, unveiling the world of oppression, that is, making it conscious; second, expulsion of the myths created and developed by the old order – this involves not only personal and professional under-standing of the influence of the old order, but also the injection of some energy to confront and challenge oneself and to take action within the system. The energy required to go against the cultural narrative is assertive energy. This also speaks to the process of self-inquiry through reflection. Reflection is a process of conscientization at differing levels; for the researcher it brings to awareness the conflict between the inner and the outer dialog, which is often suppressed within the work setting, making the private knowledge public. It also casts light on the shadow of oppression by pedagogical attitudes within the local situation in-volved in the research. The local community is also partly representa-tive of the larger political and social context and therefore any process of conscientization will have aspects which can be transferred both nationally and globally. It would seem, however, that there is the risk that conscientization itself could become oppressive when it becomes normative. For example, if conscientization becomes the dominant discourse to which everyone is persuaded to subscribe with uncritical acceptance then it runs the risk of falling into its own trap.

Transformatory learning

It has been mentioned that the cycle of reflection is a core component of the process of self-inquiry that is self as scientist (researcher/practi-tioner). The processes of reflection and action learning are also major proponents of the transformatory approach to learning (Askew and Carnell, 1998; Freshwater, 2000). Whilst in action research the focus is external, usually on professional practice within a particular context, action learning is primarily a personal activity with an internal focus (Freshwater *et al.*, 2007). Nurse teachers, like nurses, use action research in their day-to-day activity in the classroom, although it is not likely to be in a formal or conscious way. This has parallels with what Benner (1984) describes as the testing out of hypotheses in practice.

Reflecting on and evaluating teaching sessions and using this informa-tion to improve future work is utilizing some of the aspects of action research. Where this is an integral part of the teacher's daily work, teachers can feel empowered to make changes in their practice (Somekh, 1995). However, action research brings about change, not just at the group level, but also at the individual level – this could be viewed as the internal personal focus. The idea of the nurse researcher learning about the process of researching through learning in the process of carrying out research is congruent with both the action learning and the action research cycles. Reflection as transformatory education views the teacher as a learner. Askew and Carnell (1998) believe that the teacher as learner is:

> *engaged in the process of action learning and action research, reflecting on experiences, developing understanding, gaining insights into practice, making important professional judgements and bringing about actions for change.* (p. 152)

From this vantage point the teacher is not seen as a technician delivering a curriculum, but a professional learner and educator. This could be translated into nursing practice as the nurse not being seen as a technician delivering a program of care, but as an open and professional learner/educator in action. In point of fact, this is generally the case in the reality of clinical practice and as such the patient is always teaching the carer. The difficulty is that whilst this remains implicit it may result in qualified individuals feeling unable to acknowledge their limitations and ask for help (thus risking patient safety).

Healthcare research and literature is moving into a narrative space and incorporating autobiographical components to provide insight into the role, position and transformed attitude of the researcher/practitioner with regard to their role as carer (McKenzie, 2002), practitioner (Kelso, 2007) and educationalist (Esterhuizen, 2007; Freshwater, 2000; Muncey, 2000). Esterhuizen (2007), for example, reflects:

> *my process through my research has been one of combining and interrelating education, research and practice. I have not been able to distil one from the other and one aspect of my work has fed and inspired another. Understanding and exploring aspects of my own socialization have provided me with insight as to my decisions and motivations and has helped me focus my identity as a researcher and an educator. I find I am not able to provide a teaching session or conduct supervision without being aware of issues related to socialization, but I've had that for a long time. What is new to me is an awareness of personal issues that may surface and the way I now consciously deal with them – either by acknowledging them to myself and keeping them outside the dialog, or by introducing them into the discussion, if appropriate, and discussing them openly in terms of my input. From a sociological perspective, I have learned that the students participating in my study were not self-sacrificial, mindless beings adapting in order to fit in – I've seen another side. They are intelligent women, making proactive choices of how to best deal with the challenges they face and make specific decisions to reach the goal they see before them. From an educational*

perspective, facilitated reflection is immeasurably valuable, but . . . the role, input, background and history of the facilitator are vital. If the facilitator is insufficiently conscious of what is driving them as a nurse and an educator, this can alter the tool of guided reflection from being one of emancipation and empowerment to being an instrument of destruction and oppression.

Summary

Narrative has the power to change and influence. To transform. As healthcare professionals what we often do best is listen to our patients' stories and to their families. Whatever the underlying dramas of co-dependency, oppression or power may mean to us as individuals, we all have the potential to rise above it and capture our own art of caring, and in doing so form the *therapeutic I*; for we have our own story to tell and to enact. As McKenzie (2002: 35) notes:

In sharing my story I continue to construct the story of my life and in doing so construct myself. When stories are shared it creates a sense of belonging and community. This sense of belonging and of community is a powerful way of enabling us to transform self and practice, to change the story for self and others, and has a massive healing potential.

References

Allcock, N. and Standen, P. (2001) Student nurses' experiences of caring for patients in pain. *International Journal of Nursing Studies*, 38, 287–95.

Askew, S. and Carnell, E. (1998) *Transforming Learning: Individual and Global Change*. Cassell, London.

Atkins, S. and Murphy, K. (1993) Reflection: a review of the literature. *Journal of Advanced Nursing*, 18, 11–92.

Benner, P. (1984) *From Novice to Expert: Excellence and Power in Clinical Nursing Practice*. Addison-Wesley, Menlo Park, CA.

Bennett, S., Robertson, R. and Moss, P. (1992) Education: learning the pitfalls of codependency. *Nursing Management*, 25(2), 80B–80H.

Berne, E. (1991) *Games People Play*. Penguin, London.

Biering, P. (1998) 'Codependency': a disease or the root of nursing excellence? *Journal of Holistic Nursing*, 16, 320–37.

Birchenall, M. (2003) Commentary on Maria Lorentzon: Socializing nurse probationers in the late 19th and early 20th centuries – relevance of historical reflection for modern policy makers. *Nurse Education Today*, 23, 335–7.

Bishop, V. (2007) Clinical supervision: What is it? Why do we need it? in Bishop, V. (ed.) *Clinical Supervision in Practice: Essentials of Nursing Management*, 2nd edn. Palgrave Macmillan, Basingstoke, UK.

Boeree, C.G. (2006) Personality theories: Abraham Maslow. *Psychology Department: Shippensberg University.* http://www.social-psychology.de/do/pt_maslow.pdf (11 January 2007).

Bohart, A.C. (1993) Experiencing the basis of psychotherapy. *Journal of Psychotherapy Integration*, 3(1), 51–67.

Bond, M. and Holland, S. (1998) *Supervision in Context: Skills of Clinical Supervision for Nurses: A Practical Guide for Supervisees, Clinical Supervisors and Managers.* Open University Press, London.

Briant, S. and Freshwater, D. (1998) Exploring mutuality within the nurse–patient relationship. *British Journal of Nursing*, 7(4), 204–6, 208–11.

Burns, R. (1982) *Self concept development and education.* Holt Rinehart and Winston, London.

Carlson-Catalano, J. (1992) Empowering nurses for professional practice. *Nurse Outlook*, 40(3), 139–42.

Chappelle, L.S. and Sorrentino, E.A. (1993) Assessing the co-dependency issues within a nursing environment. *Nursing Management*, 24(5), 40–4.

Clare, J. (1993) A challenge to the rhetoric of emancipation: recreating a professional culture. *Journal of Advanced Nursing*, 18(7), 1033–8.

Dawson, P. (1998) The Self, in Edwards, D.S. (ed.) *Philosophical Issues in Nursing.* Macmillan, London.

Dolan, J.A., Fitzpatrick, M.L. and Herrmann, E.K. (1983) *Nursing in Society: A Historical Perspective.* W.B. Saunders Co., Philadelphia, PA.

Espeland, K. and Shanta, L. (2001) Empowering versus enabling in academia. *Journal of Nursing Education*, 40(8), 342–6.

Esterhuizen, P. (1997) *Is Experiential Learning the Link between Theory and Practice?* Contrafact, Ureterp.

Esterhuizen, P. (2007) The journey from neophyte to registered nurse – a Dutch experience. Unpublished PhD thesis. Bournemouth University, UK.

Farrell, G.A. (1997) Aggression in clinical settings: nurses' views. *Journal of Advanced Nursing*, 25(3), 501–8.

Fisher, M.L., Hinson, N. and Deets, C. (1994) Selected predictors of registered nurses' intent to stay. *Journal of Advanced Nursing*, 20(5), 950–7.

Freire, P. (1972) *Pedagogy of the Oppressed.* Penguin Books, London.

Freshwater, D. (1998) The Philosophers Stone. In Johns, C. and Freshwater, D. (eds) *Transforming nursing through reflective practice.* Blackwell Publishing, Oxford.

Freshwater, D. (2000) *Transformatory Learning in Nurse Education.* Nursing Praxis International, Southsea, UK.

Freshwater, D. (ed.) (2002) *Therapeutic Nursing: Improving Patient Care Through Self Awareness and Reflection.* Sage, London.

Freshwater, D. (2003) *Counselling Skills for Nurses, Midwives and Health Visitors.* Open University Press, Buckingham, UK.

Freshwater, D. (2007) Reflective practice and clinical supervision: two sides of the same coin? in Bishop, V. (ed.) *Clinical Supervision in Practice: Essentials of Nursing Management*, 2nd edn. Palgrave Macmillan, Basingstoke, UK.

Freshwater, D., Walsh, E. and Esterhuizen, P. (2006) Models of effective and reflective teaching and learning for best practice in clinical supervision, in V. Bishop (ed.) *Clinical Supervision in Practice: Essentials of Nursing Management*. Palgrave Macmillan, Basingstoke, UK.

Freshwater, D., Walsh, E. and Esterhuizen, P. (2007) Models of effective and reflective teaching and learning for best practice in clinical supervision, in Bishop, V. (ed.) *Clinical Supervision in Practice: Essentials of Nursing Management*, 2nd edn. Palgrave Macmillan, Basingstoke, UK.

Friedson, E. (1970) *Profession of Medicine*. Harper & Row, New York.

Glass, N. (1998) Becoming de-silenced and reclaiming voice: women speak out, in Keleher, I.I. and McInerney, P. (eds) *Nursing Matters*. Harcourt Brace & Co., Melbourne.

Greenleaf, N. (1978) The politics of self-esteem. *Nursing Digest*, 6, 1–7.

Greenwood, J. (1993) The apparent desensitization of student nurses during their professional socialization: a cognitive perspective. *Journal of Advanced Nursing*, 18(9), 1471–9.

Greenwood, J. (1998) The role of reflection in single and double loop learning. *Journal of Advanced Nursing*, 27(5), 1048–53.

Grundy, S. (1987) Critical pedagogy and the control of professional knowledge. *Discourse: Studies in the Cultural Politics of Education*, 7(2), 21–36.

Hall, S.F. and Wray, L.M. (1989) Co-dependency: nurses who give too much. *American Journal of Nursing*, November, 1456–60.

Helkama, K., Uutela, A., Pohjanheimo, E., Salminen, S., Kaponen, A. and Rantanen-Väntsi, L. (2003) Moral reasoning and values in medical school: a longitudinal study in Finland. *Scandinavian Journal of Educational Research*, 47(4), 399–411.

Holland, K. (1999) A journey to becoming: the student nurse in transition. *Journal of Advanced Nursing*, 29(1), 229–36.

Hopkins, L.M. and Jackson, W. (2002) Revisiting the issue of co-dependency in nursing: caring or caretaking? *Canadian Journal of Nursing Research*, 34(4), 35–45.

Hough, M. (1994) *A Practical Approach to Counselling*. Pitman, London.

Jacobs, M. (1988) *The Presenting Past*. Open University Press, Milton Keynes, UK.

Johns, C. (1995a) The value of reflective practice for nursing. *Journal of Clinical Nursing*, 4, 23–30.

Johns, C. (1995b) Achieving effective work as a professional activity, in Schober, J.E. and Hinchleff, S.M. (eds) *Towards Advanced Nursing Practice*. Arnold, London.

Johns, C. (1998) Caring through a reflective lens: giving meaning to being a reflective practitioner. *Nursing Inquiry*, 5, 18–24.

Jung, C.G. (1960) *The Undiscovered Self.* Routledge & Kegan Paul, London.

Kelso, R. (2007) An autoethnographic story of a gay therapist's struggle to come out of the psychodynamic closet. Unpublished Master's dissertation. Bournemouth University.

Kirby, S. (2003) Commentary on Maria Lorentzon: Socializing nurse probationers in the late 19th and early 20th centuries – relevance of historical reflection for modern policy makers. *Nurse Education Today*, 23, 332–4.

Knowles, M.S. (1980) *The Modern Practice of Adult Education: From Pedagogy to Andragogy.* Prentice-Hall, Engelwood Cliffs, NJ.

Lee, M.E. (1979) Towards better care: primary nursing. *Nursing Times*, 75(33), 133–5.

Lelean, S. (1973) *Ready for report nurse?* London: Royal College of Nursing, London. Cited in Walsh, M. and Ford, P. (1993) *Nursing Rituals: Research and Rational Actions.* Butterworth-Heinemann, Oxford.

LeRoux, R. (1978) Power, powerlessness and potential: nurses' role within the health care delivery system. *Image*, 10, 75–83.

Leyshon, S. (2002) Empowering practitioners: an unrealistic expectation of nurse education? *Journal of Advanced Nursing*, 40(4), 466–74.

Litchfield, J. (2001) Supporting nursing students who fail: a review of lecturers' practice. *Nurse Education in Practice*, 1, 142–8.

Lorentzon, M. (2003) Socializing nurse probationers in the late 19th and early 20th centuries – relevance of historical reflection for modern policy makers. *Nurse Education Today*, 23, 325–31.

MacIntosh, J. (2003) Reworking professional nursing identity. *Western Journal of Nursing Research*, 25(6), 725–41.

McKenzie, R. (2002) The importance of philosophical congruence for therapeutic use of self in practice, in Freshwater, D. (ed.) *Therapeutic Nursing: Improving Patient Care Through Self Awareness and Reflection.* Sage, London.

Maddi, S. (1989) *Personality Theories: A Comparative Analysis.* Wadsworth, Pacific Grove, CA.

Malloy, G.B. and Berkery, A.C. (1993) Co-dependency: a feminist perspective. *Journal of Psychosocial Nursing*, 31(4), 15–19.

Martsolf, D. (2002) Codependency, boundaries, and professional nurse caring: understanding differences and similarities in nursing practice. *Orthopaedic Nursing*, 21, 61–8.

Menzies-Lyth, I.E.P. (1970) *The Functioning of Social Systems as a Defence Against Anxiety.* Tavistock, London.

Menzies-Lyth, I.E.P. (1988) *Containing Anxiety in Institutions: Selected Essays.* Free Association Books, London.

Mezirow, J. (1975) *Education for Perspective Transformation: Women's Re-Entry Programs in Community Colleges.* Center for Adult Development, Teachers College, Columbia University, New York.

Mezirow, J. (1981) A critical theory of adult learning and education. *Adult Education*, 32(1), 3–24.

Mullins, L. (1989) *Management and Organisational Behaviour*, 2nd edn. Pitman, London.

Muncey, T. (2000) The good nurse: born or made? Unpublished PhD thesis. Cranfield University.

Nåden, D. and Eriksson, K. (2000) The phenomenon of confirmation: an aspect of nursing as an art. *International Journal for Human Caring*, 4(3), 23–8.

Nåden, D. and Eriksson, K. (2002) Encounter: a fundamental category of nursing as an art. *International Journal for Human Caring*, 6(1), 34–40.

Nåden, D. and Eriksson, K. (2004) Understanding the importance of values and moral attitudes in nursing care in preserving human dignity. *Nursing Science Quarterly*, 17(1), 86–91.

Newman, M. (1994) *Health as Expanding Consciousness*. National League for Nursing Press, New York.

Parse, R.R. (1987) *Nursing Science: Major Paradigms, Theories, and Critiques*. W.B. Saunders, Philadelphia, PA.

Priest, S. (1991) *Theories of the mind*. Houghton and Miffin, Boston.

Randle, J. (2003) Bullying in the nursing profession. *Journal of Advanced Nursing*, 43(4), 395–401.

Roberts, S.J. (1983) Oppressed group behaviour: implications for nursing. *Advances in Nursing Science*, 5, 21–30.

Rogers, C.R. (1991) *Client-Centered Therapy*. Constable, London.

Rogers, M.E. (1970) *An Introduction to the Theoretical Basis of Nursing*. F.A. Davis Co., Philadephia, PA.

Rotter, J.B. (1966) Generalized expectancies for internal versus external control of reinforcement. *Psychological Monographs*, 80(609), 1–28.

Rotter, J.B. (1971) External control and internal control. *Psychology Today*, 5, 37–59.

Schön, D.A. (1983) *The Reflective Practitioner: How Professionals Think in Action*. Basic Books, New York.

Scott, I. (1998) Challenging the future. *Nursing Management*, 4(9), 18–21.

Sherman, J.B., Cardea, J.M., Gaskill, S.D. and Tynan, C.M. (1989) Caring: commitment to excellence or condemnation to conformity? *Journal of Psychosocial Nursing*, 27(8), 25–9.

Smith, P. and Gray, B. (2001a) Reassessing the concept of emotional labour in student nurse education: role of link lecturers and mentors in a time of change. *Nurse Education Today*, 21, 230–7.

Smith, P. and Gray, B. (2001b) Emotional labour of nursing revisited: caring and learning 2000. *Nurse Education in Practice*, 1, 42–9.

Somekh, B. (1995) The contribution of action research to development in social endeavours: A position paper on action research methodology. *British Educational Research Journal*, 21(3), 339–55.

Spencer, D.G. (1986) Employee voice and employee retention. *Academy of Management Journal*, 29, 488–502.

Spouse, J. (2001) Workplace learning: pre-registration nursing students' perspectives. *Nurse Education in Practice*, 1, 149–56.

Stein, L.I. (1967) The doctor–nurse game. *Archives of General Psychiatry*, 16, 699–703.

Stein, L. (1978) The doctor–nurse game, in Dingwall, R. and McIntosh, J. (eds) *Readings in the Sociology of Nursing*. Churchill Livingstone, Edinburgh.

Stein, L., Watts, D. and Howell, T. (1990) The doctor–nurse game revisited. *New England Journal of Medicine*, 322, 546–9.

Stickley, T. and Freshwater, D. (2002) The art of loving and the therapeutic relationship. *Nursing Inquiry*, 9(4), 250–6.

Taylor, S., White, B. and Muncer, S. (1999) Nurses' cognitive structural models of work-based stress. *Journal of Advanced Nursing*, 29(4), 974–83.

Watson, J. (1988) *Nursing: Human Science and Human Care – A Theory of Nursing*. National League for Nursing Press, New York.

Watson, R., Deary, I.J. and Lea, A. (1999) A longitudinal study into the perceptions of caring and nursing among student nurses. *Journal of Advanced Nursing*, 29(5), 1228–37.

Widdershoven, G.A.M. (1999) Care, cure and interpersonal understanding. *Journal of Advanced Nursing*, 29(5), 1163–9.

Wilbur, K. (1981) *Up from Eden. A transpersonal view of human evolution*. Routledge, London.

Wilson, A. and Startup, R. (1991) Nurse socialization: issues and problems. *Journal of Advanced Nursing*, 16, 1478–86.

Wright, S.G. (1994) *My Patient – My Nurse: The Practice of Primary Nursing*, 2nd edn. Scutari Press, London.

Yates, J.G. and McDaniel, J.L. (1994) Are you losing yourself in codependency? *American Journal of Nursing*, April, 32–6.

Chapter 9

Developing a reflective curriculum

Philip Esterhuizen, Dawn Freshwater and Gwen Sherwood

Introduction

In 2000 the WHO (Europe) published a declaration stating the importance of developing intra- and interdisciplinary education programs at undergraduate and postgraduate levels. The rationale behind this statement was to promote cooperative and interdisciplinary working to improve patient care (WHO, 2000). In the United Kingdom interprofessional education approaches have focussed on generic issues influencing the disciplines. It has, however, also supported the development of innovations to increase and utilize practice as a learning environment, particularly as it reflects the varied and complex situation of healthcare provision (ENB and DH, 2001). Similar initiatives have been proposed and developed internationally, with generic and core training being suggested in both Australia and the USA.

In Europe and specifically in the Netherlands two documents have been instrumental in influencing nursing. The first is a new professional code of practice,[1] which implicitly outlines a humanistic philosophy carrying implications for patient care and staff. The second document is an educational report[2] which provides guidelines for educational and clinical settings regarding future nursing programs.

---

[1] *Beroepsprofiel van de Verpleegkundige* (Leistra *et al.*, 1999)
[2] *Gekwalificeerd voor de Toekomst* (Commissie Kwalificatiestructuur, 1996)

In the Republic of Ireland, government policy underpins the need (a) for an integrated, interdisciplinary response to health needs, (b) to develop a culture that supports health research, and (c) to support staff development (Department of Health and Children, 2001a, b; Government of Ireland, 2006). In specific relation to nursing and midwifery, there is the need to provide education that enables the development of specialist and advanced knowledge and skills (Government of Ireland, 1998). These suggestions have been supported by recommendations of the National Council for Professional Development of Nursing and Midwifery (2004a, b, c, 2005a, b).

The focus of global and governmental initiatives to develop person-centered care from an interprofessional perspective has also been addressed and is becoming more visible through the increase in nursing research underpinning similar approaches (Clark, 2005; Esterhuizen, 1997, 2007; MacNeil and Evans, 2005; Schoenhofer, 2001; Sumner and Danielson, 2007; Walsh *et al.*, 2007). In terms of curriculum development a person-centered and interprofessional approach needs to be supported by an educational psychology that shows clear links between the organizational philosophies directing care and education. In other words, there should be a logical connection and correlation between the philosophy of care and the philosophy of (clinical) education. This approach has far-reaching implications for the collaboration between institutions providing care and those providing education.

Nursing is based on a philosophy of care incorporating *personalized care* and *professional treatment* focussed on the *individual,* whereby their specific needs and problems are taken into account. This approach demands the nurse's ability to enter into a collaborative relationship with the patient based on his/her own knowledge and skill if the relationship is to result in patient-centeredness. The nurse's knowledge and skill should be founded on sound systematic and critical thinking. In other words he/she should be able to critically appraise nursing interventions and outcomes. In short: an expert and autonomous professional able to reflect-in- and on-action. *Education* of nursing students – in both the academic and clinical environments – should strive for the *individual's development and personal growth*. This will result in an inquiring, questioning attitude, greater motivation and work satisfaction, and a positive attitude to lifelong learning. *Student support* should, therefore, be mirrored in a philosophy of mentorship and guidance. Systematic mentorship should take specific characteristics of individual students into account, be sensitive to their needs and problems and contextualize the support in terms of the student's seniority.

Identifying the need for students to be supported and nurtured in their development does not exclude the necessity for critical and meaningful assessment. The UK's Nursing and Midwifery Council (1999, 2002a, 2004, 2007) has, in various documents, stipulated levels of practice required by nurses and the expectations of mentors. However Duffy (2003) and Scholes and Albarran (2005) have highlighted the fact that mentors in practice settings are not always comfortable or expert enough to negatively assess students. In Chapter 8 reference was made to work by Espeland and Shanta (2001), Smith and Gray (2001) and Spouse (2001a) regarding interdependence between student and faculty which could result in discomfort and a conflict of loyalties in terms of assessment.

In order to respond to the continually changing dynamic of health-care, educational programs need to be innovative and flexible. To achieve this, it is essential that there is collaborative engagement between the academic and clinical settings. A collaboration of this nature and magnitude is a major challenge considering the diversity of underpinning beliefs, perceptions and practices. Collective critical reflection (Freire, 1972) (see Chapter 8) is, therefore, essential to bridge the gap between practice and education (Campbell *et al.*, 1994; Freshwater, 1998a; Mallik, 1993; Rolfe, 1998; Rolfe *et al.*, 2001) – we would argue that developing a curriculum based on reflective practice and reflexivity is one way of achieving this outcome.

Competency-based education

Although there appears to be a move towards patient-centered care and the awareness for more reflective components within the curriculum, the reality is that competency-based education is the approach most generally incorporated in nursing education. All the national documents[3] studied focus on qualifications and competencies of some form or another but, although nomenclature is not standardized, the discussion addresses two concepts: qualifications and competencies.

---

[3] *Gekwalificeerd voor de Toekomst* (Commissie Kwalificatiestructuur, 1996)
Framework for the Establishment of Clinical Nurse/Midwife Specialist Posts Intermediate Pathway (National Council for the Professional Development of Nursing and Midwifery, 2004b)
Framework for the Establishment of Advanced Nurse Practitioner and Advanced Midwife Practitioner Posts (National Council for the Professional Development of Nursing and Midwifery, 2004c)
Standards of proficiency for pre-registration nursing education (Nursing and Midwifery Council, 2004).

Dutch authors Peschar and Wesselingh (1995) describe *qualifications* as being preparation in a broad spectrum of skills for a profession, where there is reference to an external curriculum. In contrast they describe *competencies* as the knowledge, skills and attitude an individual has developed in a variety of areas, where it concerns abstract values such as critical thinking, problem solving and communication skills. In short, it is the ability to carry out an activity without it being dictated by external criteria.

In contrast, Watson *et al.* (2002) cite McClelland (1973) as suggesting competence being an alternative to intelligence for certain jobs – skills being the requirements for the job at hand, rather than academic prowess. Prior to discussing the definition more fully, the ideas behind using competencies and competency frameworks should be looked at more closely.

From an educational perspective competencies are used to provide (a) the recognition of learning and (b) links between the individual and organizational requirements. Ultimately this is designed to deliver qualified staff members, fit for practice in various healthcare areas, which are able to function independently and without supervision. With regard to qualified staff, Storey *et al.* (2002) list a number of uses for competency frameworks, including providing clarity of the role and responsibilities of the professional in order to protect the public and promote accountability. Watson *et al.* (2002) describe competencies and occupational standards as being 'flip sides of the same coin' and suggest that, while competencies specify what an individual is expected to do, the occupational standards specify what the public may expect.

The idea of clarity regarding the nursing role is supported by the document *Defining Nursing* by the UK's Royal College of Nursing (RCN, 2003) and the Nursing and Midwifery Council's *Code of Professional Conduct* (NMC, 2002b). They provide general behavioral and attitudinal competencies informing and clarifying the nurse's role to those both in and out of the profession. The specific competency frameworks as developed by the NMC (2003) also aim to protect the public from inferior practice by setting minimal standards for professional functioning. The NMC link their specific competency frameworks to the *Code of Professional Conduct*.

In contrast to the way Watson *et al.* (2002) describe occupational standards as being a safeguard for the public, the Skills for Health (2003) document describes the instrument primarily in terms of learning and quality improvement. This is also true for the Knowledge and

Skills Framework (DH, 2003), but this framework links the idea of personal development to a system of review and remuneration.

Reflective practice

As discussed throughout this book, the ability to reflect on experience is an essential aspect of learning. Reflective practice is, however, more than simply asking why, it is not a new concept and has influenced nursing education extensively in the past decades.

Palmer *et al.* (1994: 2) refer to Street (1991) and suggest that reflection in nursing can be seen as a way for nurses to become completely aware:

> *Empower nurses to become fully cognizant of their own knowledge and actions, the personal and professional histories which have shaped them, the symbols and metaphors which sustain them in practice, their nursing experiences, and the potentialities and constraints of their work setting.*

Professionals need more than purely empirical knowledge to be competent as a nurse and in the past 20 years it has been shown that reflection is an instrument by which to learn from practice situations. Reflection in nursing can be seen as part of the developmental process of a nurse – through learning at different levels – to become a critical, autonomous practitioner capable of meeting the needs of the individual patients. (These issues have been developed further to include therapeutic use of self in Chapter 8.) The concept of learning at different levels – single, double and triple loop learning (Fig. 9.1) (Freshwater, 1998; Lingsma and Scholten, 2001) – has been referred to in Chapter 5 and so will not be discussed in detail again. However, it is important to acknowledge that reflective thinking in nursing practice is often applied at the first two levels, but it should not be ignored that nurses in practice are confronted with numerous ethical questions that can and should be addressed at the third level.

It is also important to pause briefly in order to clarify that reflection-in-action which occurs while practicing influences the decisions made and care given, and reflection-on-action, which occurs retrospectively, contributes to the development of practice skills (Palmer *et al.*, 1994; Schön, 1991).

To enable the practitioner to learn from reflection-in- and on-action it is essential that the practice setting is safe, organized and structured, not relying on ad hoc learning. These three aspects, together with education,

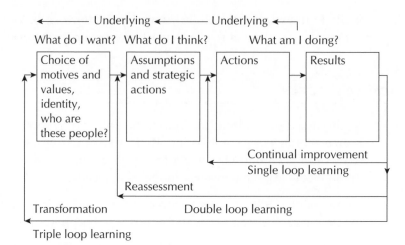

Figure 9.1 Transformational learning (Lingsma and Scholten, 2001: 55).

support, mentorship, leadership and the operationalization of a learning climate are the preconditions for lifelong learning using work-related experiences. According to Palmer *et al.* (1994: 13):

> *Practitioners learn from both types of reflection and these need to be facilitated within a practice-led curriculum. Learning by reflection can be facilitated most effectively within a practicum.*

The suggestion by Palmer *et al.* (1994) is, therefore, that reflection should be facilitated by someone who is an expert in nursing, and also expert in the art of reflection and its facilitation. Mentors, clinical educators, lecturer-practitioners and the various titles of advanced nurses could all have active roles in promoting reflection, reflective practice and reflexivity (Daloz, 1986). Figure 9.2 illustrates the mutual dependence between challenge and support and suggests that mentors should focus on supporting, challenging and providing a philosophy.

The role Daloz puts forward as being mentorship is, two decades later, synonomous with that held by facilitators of reflection. In order to achieve the support, challenge and philosophical elements, and based on Daloz's (1986) suggestion, the following skills are needed:

Support

- Listening skills
- Ability to provide structure
- Ability to articulate positive expectations
- Willingness and ability to defend the learner's best interests

- Willingness to share ideas and experiences
- Ability to make the learning experience special for the learner.

Challenge

- Set assignments
- Articulate opposing points of view
- Set high expectations
- Present hypotheses
- Become involved in discussions.

With respect to challenging learners, it is important that the facilitators be aware of the timing of the challenge, the atmosphere of collaboration, the skill and ability to take calculated risks and be sensitive to their communication skills and way in which the challenge is presented.

Philosophy

- The environment should include the support and challenge to facilitate learning.
- The facilitator is the guide providing direction and methods for reflection and learning.

In Chapter 6 we referred to the interrelationship between reflection, reflective practice and clinical supervision and from the reality of educational and clinical practice it will be clear that the preconditions for

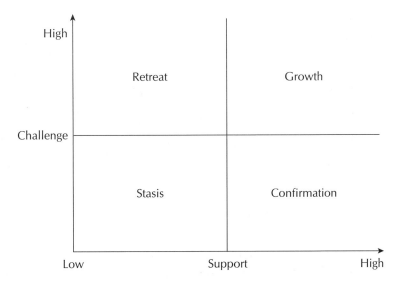

Figure 9.2 Mutually dependent relationships in mentoring (Palmer *et al.,* 1994: 38).

a reflective practice do not spontaneously arise, nor are they automatically sustainable. It is also not automatically a fact that practice-based mentors will have the facilitative skills to support reflection. This has a direct inpact on mentor preparation which should include preparing them to work directly with learners in identified situations, feel comfortable with posing questions while working in the clinical or educational setting and have knowledge and ideas that can be measured and validated in practice.

Elsewhere in this book (Chapters 5 and 6) extensive reference is made to issues of power and empowerment. Although written more than a decade ago, DeMarco's (1993: 1245) work places the concept of empowerment within a mentorship framework. She describes empowerment as an *internal awakening in which a trusted mentor acts as an encourager of untapped abilities*. DeMarco also suggests that empowerment is a way *to increase another's self-confidence through solicitation of tangible productive acts which are deemed 'successful.'* This discussion also highlights the question whether empowerment could be seen as assuming a masculine paradigm of success to exercise control over others – a concept discussed in detail in Chapter 5. But within the framework of reflective practice in which mentorship and facilitated reflection are important concepts, methods of empowerment are important issues to take into account.

Reflective curriculum

It is clear from the discussion in this chapter and elsewhere in this book that a reflective curriculum needs to be based on a sound educational philosophy that operationalizes the principles of caring, empowerment and emancipation and aspires to develop the student as a lifelong learner. This approach requires strong collaboration between clinical and academic partners in order to stimulate and develop opportunities for learning and professional development.

The principal aim of a reflective curriculum is to develop and support an environment in which learning from and through practice results from the individual bringing together of self-knowledge, expertise at work and formal knowledge (Flanagan *et al.*, 2000). This will be instrumental in nurturing and developing the highest standards of professional practice.

Fundamental to a reflective curriculum is the collaboration between the academic and clinical settings and the student. Within the practice-based learning model, while generic theoretical and practice principles

are identified within the prescribed program curriculum, it is important that the learner is supported and facilitated, allowing the individual
to develop a personal line of inquiry, draw on their existing knowledge
and identify their individual learning needs in relation to their practice.
This can be achieved within a group or in individual assignments. To
support teamworking, each student should be expected to negotiate and
achieve practice learning outcomes that fit their individual requirements,
those of their practice and their program.

Inquiry-based learning (Kahn and O'Rourke, 2005) can be used to encourage learning from practice and experience. This approach to
learning is an active educational approach relying on facilitative teaching methods and carrying an expectation that the learner construct their
own knowledge by engaging in supported processes of inquiry, often
achieved through groupwork. Using this approach, learners draw upon
the reality of their work-related experience to enter and engage in the
process of inquiry (Clarke and Wilcockson, 2001; Litchfield, 1999;
Lloyd Jones, 2005; Penney and Warelow, 1999; Spouse, 2001b). Using
inquiry-based learning three levels of knowledge inform the inquiry
process: knowledge-in-use, knowledge-in-waiting and evidenced-based
knowing. Through this process the learner can relate newly learned
theoretical principles, evidence and skills to their practice and, so,
develop their expertise. Learners are encouraged and supported to take
responsibility, and learning can take place via lectures, seminars and
tutorials, groupwork, self-directed and supported learning and portfolio development. The most important objective of this approach is to
create and sustain a negotiated relationship between practice and education in order to support the development of a nursing and healthcare
workforce capable of adapting to a changing healthcare environment,
stimulate sustainable lifelong learners and achieve the competencies
demanded by professional organizations and stakeholders.

While theoretical and practice principles are identified and delivered
in the program, there should be designated academic and clinical
supervisors to support and facilitate the individual's learning process
by identifying individual learning needs in relation to practice. Clinical
supervision is a key process to enabling practitioners to translate their
experiential knowledge into learning (see Chapter 6) as is reflective
journaling, narrating experiences and portfolio development (see
Chapters 5 and 11).

Within a reflective curriculum, while a substantial percentage of assessment takes place in the clinical setting, it simultaneously poses many
challenges: namely, the ethical aspect of involvement in a nurse/patient

relationship; the morals of evaluation within the principles of reflection-in-action and on-action; the objective/subjective measurement of practice and the resultant observer bias inherent in such a system.

The objective for each learner is to achieve integration of theory and practice, develop ability, competence and expertise in their profession, and develop an approach to lifelong learning and an attitude for continuing professional development. Assessing this level of abstraction poses challenges, and while assessment has a role in verifying that appropriate learning has taken place it is important to ensure that the methods of assessment are not a method of punishment, but an aid to learning, providing opportunities for personal development, critical reflection and skills development (see also Chapter 11). It is essential that assessments reflect the principles of learning from practice and integrating theory. As such, each assessment should include documentation of how the learner has achieved theory/practice integration and all assignments should be graded by an academic and the clinical supervisor. There should, ideally, be opportunities for self-assessment as this fosters a (self-)critical approach in the individual. Methods of continuous assessment could include essays, case studies, skills-based assessment, computer-based learning and assessment exercises, nurse/patient assessment and the development of a clinical/work portfolio which could incorporate aspects of a 360-degree feedback.

Journaling and portfolios may provide documentary assessment allowing learners to present evidence of critical thinking and clinical performance and provide a medium for them to use this experience for reflection and learning.

In the practicum

Practical implications of a reflective curriculum are sometimes difficult to visualize. We close this chapter with an example of a reflective approach to teaching and learning. The following vignette is presented as an example of how elements of a reflective curriculum could be operationalized. In this case, during the first year of a four-year Bachelor's education, students have practical placements as follows: one three-day orientation prior to starting with the theoretical components of the program, two two-week placements and one ten-week placement.

Objectives

The objectives of these placements are:

(1) Integration of theory and practice:
  - Developing competence of already learned skills in 'real' situations.
  - Provide the student with the opportunity of staying in contact with the reality of the hospital.
  - Provide the student with practice experience as a framework to use for the theory provided in the academic setting.
(2) Provide the student with the opportunity of more contact with the practice setting before the more lengthy placements.

Buildup of the placements

(1) The students have various contact moments with the practice setting:
  - one three-day orientation prior to starting with the theoretical components of the course,
  - one two-week placement at the end of the first study block,
  - one two-week placement at the end of the second study block,
  - one ten-week placement in the fourth study block.
(2) The tests of competencies related to the three placements are cumulative – the competencies relating to personal and basic nursing care are always evaluated in all situations.
(3) The placement consists of a 36-hour week.

Mentorship during the orientation placement

The students are invited by letter to the three-day orientation and are requested to complete an assignment as preparation.

Day 1

Assignment (1) 'What are your thoughts, feelings and expectations when you think of your first day in placement in the hospital?'

On the first day of the orientation, the hospital-based educator meets the student in the hospital in the morning and the group starts with a round of meeting each other using assignment 1 if desired. All the assignments are discussed with the students. The hospital-based educator must ensure that all students have the opportunity to share their experiences with the group, taking into account that the students do not yet know each other.

In the course of the day, the students attend an observation workshop (see assignment 2, below) and then discuss their experiences

Table 9.1 Example form for completion by students during observation workshop.

Objective information	Subjective information	Personal reactions
How do you find the ward/unit? (Describe what you find, using your five senses and the following cues) What do you see? What do you hear? What is the staff doing? What does the staff look like? What does the staff say?	What do you think is happening on the unit/ward? Who are the people you see? Are there things happening you've seen before, or are there things happening that are new to you?	Describe your reaction to what you see. Which thoughts, feelings, emotions and sensations are you experiencing?
Comments	Comments	Comments

(assignment 3), interpret them (assignment 4) and reflect on the day (assignment 5).

The students are introduced on the ward where they will be placed and the hospital-based educator ensures that the ward/unit is informed ahead of time. The ward/unit provides a mentor for the student and ideally the student should have the same mentor for the second and third days of the orientation.

Assignment (2) 'Observation workshop'

Using a printed form (Table 9.1) which allows for observations and comments, the student notes down their observations of people and activities during the 90 minutes on the ward/unit.

On completion of the observation workshop they move to assignment 3.

Assignment (3) 'Write up your experiences of the observation workshop'

The students discuss their experiences of the observation workshop in the group/small groups. They are required to describe their feelings relating to the workshop, the behavior of the registered staff, and their ideas of the professional role within the hospital.

Assignment (4) 'What is your philosophy/vision of care?'

Using a variety of pictures, students are required to choose a maximum of two pictures symbolizing their philosophy/vision of care. They write up their interpretation of 'care' and share it with the group.

Assignment (5) 'What are your thoughts, feelings and experiences as you look back on your first day in the hospital?'

The first day of the orientation is ended with a reflective session. The students share their reflections on their first impressions, feelings and emotions and the role these have/have had on their behavior. The students are encouraged to write short notes for themselves.

Outputs

The students hand in all the products from assignments 1–5 to their hospital-based educator. With students' consent the assignments are copied and form part of their portfolios for the rest of their education. The rationale is that the assignments form the basis for the development of the students' professional philosophy and are referred to throughout the rest of the four-year program. Students are encouraged to reflect on changes in their personal philosophy.

Day 2

In preparation for day 2, the students write up their thoughts, feelings and expectations in anticipation of their first experience with patients.

They are met by the hospital-based educator early in the morning, provided with uniforms and delivered to the ward/unit. They work a full day duty with an appointed mentor (Registered Nurse or senior student). The hospital-based educator is available via a bleep the full day and looks in on the students throughout the day to follow progress.

Day 3

In preparation for day 3, students make notes of their experiences on day 2.

The students are met in the morning by the hospital-based educator and they share their experiences of day 2 with the group in a plenary session (the mentors from the wards/units are not present).

The students' assignments 1–5 are returned to them and, in small groups, they reflect on the past three days using their assignments.

In the afternoon the students use their reflections from the morning sessions to formulate learning objectives for (a) the theoretical program and (b) their first two-week placement.

Preparation at school for the placement

Approximately a week before the start of each placement, the hospital-based educator provides information on the practice placement and explains how competencies will be evaluated. The students are encouraged to set up learning objectives in preparation for their placement.

Mentorship during the practical placements

The hospital-based educator meets the students on the first day of the placement to organize practical aspects of the placements such as uniforms and badges.

- During a plenary session the students are supported in (a) setting up learning objectives for the placement (also using their evaluations from the third orientation day), (b) formulating their expectations of the placement and (c) setting out a plan of action.
- The students are escorted to the ward/unit (the same unit where they did their orientation, whenever possible).
- An afternoon meeting is held with the students and their named mentors (or a representative from the ward/unit).
  - The hospital-based educator provides an explanation of the placement and which set objectives need to be achieved.
  - The students allocated to a specific ward/unit meet with the mentor/representative to discuss expectations.
  - The students write a short report of the expectations which is signed by the student and the ward mentor/representative.

During the two-week placements no formal midway evaluation is held unless problems arise. During the third, 10-week, placement a formal midway evaluation is held between the student, mentor and hospital-based educator. During the placement the hospital-based educator drops in on the student in the ward to answer questions and discuss possible problems with the student and/or mentor.

A final evaluation of the placement occurs on the last working day of the placement. Each student is responsible for having the evaluation documentation filled out with the ward/unit-based mentor prior to coming to the evaluation meeting. The mentors are not present during this meeting. The students hand in a report in which they describe their learning process during the placement, how and whether they achieved their personal objectives, and reflect on their vision/philosophy of care. During the evaluation the students look back on their current placement and set learning objectives for the next one. The hospital-based educator feeds back any relevant information from the final evaluation to the ward/unit.

Summary

While a substantial percentage of assessment in a reflective curriculum takes place in the clinical setting it, simultaneously, poses many challenges. The challenges include the ethical aspect of involvement in a nurse–patient relationship; the morals of evaluation within the principles of reflection-in-action and on-action; the objective/subjective measurement of practice and the resultant observer bias inherent in such a system.

Each learner's objectives are to integrate theory and practice, develop ability, competence and expertise in their profession, develop an approach to lifelong learning and an attitude for continuing professional development. Assessing this level of abstraction poses challenges and, while assessment has a role in verifying that appropriate learning has taken place, it is important to ensure that the methods of assessment are not a method of punishment, but an aid to learning, providing opportunities for personal development, critical reflection and skills development (see also Chapter 11). It is essential that assessments reflect the principles of learning from practice and integrating theory. As such, each assessment should include documentation of how the learner has achieved theory/practice integration and all assignments should be graded by an academic and the clinical supervisor. There should, ideally, be opportunities for self-assessment as this fosters a (self-)critical approach in the individual. Methods of continuous assessment could include essays, case studies, skills-based assessment, computer-based learning and assessment exercises, nurse/patient assessment and the development of a clinical/work portfolio which could incorporate aspects of a 360-degree feedback.

Journaling and portfolios provide documentary assessment, allowing learners to present evidence of critical thinking and clinical performance, and provide a medium for them to use this experience for reflection and learning.

References

Campbell, I.E., Larivee, L., Field, P.A., Day, R.A. and Reutter, L. (1994) Learning to nurse in the clinical setting. *Journal of Advanced Nursing*, 20, 1125–31.

Clark, C.S. (2005) Transforming Nursing Education: A Partnership Social System for Alignment with Philosophies of Care. *International Journal of Nursing Education Scholarship*. (http://www.bepress.com/cgi/viewcontent. cgi?article=1100&context=ijnes)

Clarke, C.L. and Wilcoxon, J. (2001) Professional and organizational learning: analyzing the relationship with the development of practice. *Journal of Advanced Nursing*, 34(2), 264–72.

Commissie Kwalificatiestructuur (1996) *Gekwalificeerd voor de Toekomst*. Zoetermeer/Rijswijk, Ministerie van Onderwijs, Cultuur en Wetenschappen/ Ministerie van Volksgezondheid, Welzijn en Sport.

Daloz, L.A. (1986) *Effective Mentoring and Teaching: Realizing the Transformational Power of Adult Learning Experiences*. Jossey-Bass, San Francisco.

DeMarco, R. (1993) Mentorship: a feminist critique of current research. *Journal of Advanced Nursing*, 18, 1242–50.

Department of Health and Children (2001a) *Quality and Fairness: A Health System for You*. Department of Health and Children, Dublin, Republic of Ireland.

Department of Health and Children (2001b) *Making Knowledge Work for Health: A Strategy for Health Research*. Department of Health and Children, Dublin, Republic of Ireland.

DH (Department of Health) (2003) *The NHS Knowledge and Skills Framework (NHS KSF) and Development Review Guidance – Working Draft*. www.doh.gov.uk/thenhsksf

Duffy, K. (2003) *Failing students: a qualitative study of factors that influence the decisions regarding the assessment of students' competence to practice*. Nursing and Midwifery Council website (http://www.nmc-uk.org/ aFrameDisplay.aspx?DocumentID=1329).

ENB and DH (English Nursing Board and Department of Health) (2001) *Placements in Focus: Guidance for Education in Practice and Health Care Professions*. English Nursing Board, London.

Espeland, K. and Shanta, L. (2001) Empowering versus enabling in academia. *Journal of Nursing Education*, 40(8), 342–6.

Esterhuizen, P. (1997) *Is Experiential Learning the Link between Theory and Practice?* Contrafact, Ureterp.

Esterhuizen, P. (2007) The journey from neophyte to registered nurse – a Dutch experience. Unpublished PhD thesis. Bournemouth University, UK.

Flanagan, J., Baldwin, S. and Clarke, D. (2000) Work-based learning as a means of developing and assessing nursing competence. *Journal of Clinical Nursing*, 9, 360–8.

Freire, P. (1972) *Pedagogy of the Oppressed*. Penguin Books, London.

Freshwater, D. (1998) The Philosopher's Stone, in Johns, C. and Freshwater, D. (eds) *Transforming Nursing through Reflective Practice*. Blackwell Science, Oxford.

Government of Ireland (1998) *Report of the Commission on Nursing: A blueprint for the future*. The Stationery Office, Dublin.

Government of Ireland (2006) *Report of the National Task Force on Medical Staffing*. The Stationery Office, Dublin.

Kahn, P. and O'Rourke, K. (2005) Understanding enquiry-based learning, in Barrett, T., MacLabhrainn, I. and Fallon, H. (eds) *Handbook of Enquiry and Problem Based Learning: Irish Case Studies and International Perspective*. Centre for Excellence in Learning and Teaching, National University of Ireland, Galway, Ireland (http://www.nuigalway.ie/celt/pblbook/) (downloaded November 6, 2007).

Leistra, E., Liefhebber, S., Geomini, M. and Hens, H. (1999) *Beroepsprofiel van de Verpleegkundige*. Elsevier/De Tijdstroom, Utrecht, Netherlands.

Lingsma, M. and Scholten, M. (2001) *Coachen op Competentieontwikkeling*. Uitgeverij Nelissen, Soest, Netherlands.

Litchfield, M. (1999) Practice wisdom. *Advances in Nursing Science*, 22(2), 62–73.

Lloyd Jones, M. (2005) Role development and effective practice in specialist and advanced practice roles in acute hospital settings: systematic review and meta-synthesis. *Journal of Advanced Nursing*, 49(2), 191–209.

McClelland, D.C. (1973) Testing for competence rather than for intelligence. *American Psychologist*, 28, 1–14.

MacNeil, M.S. and Evans, M. (2005) The pedagogy of caring in nursing education. *International Journal for Human Caring*, 9(4), 45–51.

Mallik, M. (1993) Theory to practice links. *Senior Nurse*, 13(4), 41–6.

National Council for the Professional Development of Nursing and Midwifery (2004a) *Report of the Continuing Professional Development of Staff Nurses and Midwives*. National Council for the Professional Development of Nursing and Midwifery, Dublin, Republic of Ireland.

National Council for the Professional Development of Nursing and Midwifery (2004b) *Framework for the Establishment of Clinical Nurse/ Midwife Specialist Posts Intermediate Pathway*, 2nd edn. National Council for the Professional Development of Nursing and Midwifery, Dublin, Republic of Ireland.

National Council for the Professional Development of Nursing and Midwifery (2004c) *Framework for the Establishment of Advanced Nurse Practitioner and Advanced Midwife Practitioner Posts*, 2nd edn. National Council for the Professional Development of Nursing and Midwifery, Dublin, Republic of Ireland.

National Council for the Professional Development of Nursing and Midwifery (2005a) *An Evaluation of the Extent and Nature of Nurse-Led/ Midwife-Led Services in Ireland*. National Council for the Professional Development of Nursing and Midwifery, Dublin, Republic of Ireland.

National Council for the Professional Development of Nursing and Midwifery (2005b) *Agenda for the Future Professional Development of Public Health Nursing*. National Council for the Professional Development of Nursing and Midwifery, Dublin, Republic of Ireland.

NMC (Nursing and Midwifery Council) (1999) *Fitness for Practice*. UKCC Commission for Nursing and Midwifery Education, London.

NMC (Nursing and Midwifery Council) (2002a) *Standards for the preparation of teachers of nursing and midwifery*. NMC, London.

NMC (Nursing and Midwifery Council) (2002b) *Code of Professional Conduct* (http://www.nmc-uk.org/nmc/main/publications/codeOfProfessional-
Conduct.pdf).

NMC (Nursing and Midwifery Council) (2003) Third part of the new register:
specialist community public health nursing. Proposed competency framework. Consultation background information (www.nmc-uk.org/nmc/main/
consultation).

NMC (Nursing and Midwifery Council) (2004) *Standards of proficiency for
pre-registration nursing education*. NMC, London.

NMC (Nursing and Midwifery Council) (2007) *Mentors need to learn to fail
nurses* (http://www.nmc-uk.org/aArticle.aspx?ArticleID=1256).

Palmer, A., Burns, S. and Bulman, C. (1994) *Reflective Practice in Nursing:
The Growth of the Professional Practitioner*. Blackwell Science, Oxford.

Penney, W. and Warelow, J. (1999) Understanding the prattle of praxis.
Nursing Inquiry, 6, 259–68.

Peschar, J.L. and Wesselingh, A. (1995) *Onderwijssociologie*, 1st edn.
Wolters-Noordhoff, Groningen.

RCN (Royal College of Nursing) (2003) Defining Nursing: Nursing is . . .
(http://www.rcn.org.uk/downloads/definingnursing/definingnursing-a5.pdf).

Rolfe, G. (1998) *Expanding the Theory–Practice Gap*. Butterworth
Heinemann, Oxford.

Rolfe, G., Freshwater, D. and Jasper, M. (2001) *Critical Reflection for Nursing
and the Helping Professions: A User's Guide*. Palgrave, Basingstoke, UK.

Schoenhofer, S.O. (2001) Infusing the nursing curriculum with literature on
caring: an idea whose time has come. *International Journal for Human
Caring*, 5(2), 7–14.

Scholes, J. and Albarran, J. (2005) Failure to fail: facing the consequences of
inaction. *Nursing in Critical Care*, 10(3), 113–15.

Schön, D. (1991) *The Reflective Practitioner*, 2nd edn. Jossey-Bass, San
Francisco.

Skills for Health (2003) *Information briefing 1–8* (http://www.skills-
forhealth.org.uk).

Smith, P. and Gray, B. (2001) Emotional labour of nursing revisited: caring
and learning 2000. *Nurse Education in Practice*, 1, 42–9.

Spouse, J. (2001a) Workplace learning: pre-registration nursing students'
perspectives. *Nurse Education in Practice*, 1, 149–56.

Spouse, J. (2001b) Bridging theory and practice in the supervisory relationship: a sociocultural perspective. *Journal of Advanced Nursing*, 33(4),
512–22.

Storey, L., Howard, J. and Gillies, A. (2002) *Competency in Healthcare: A
Practical Guide to Competency Frameworks*. Radcliffe Medical Press,
London.

Street, A. (1991) *From Image to Action: Reflection in Nursing Practice*.
Deakin University, Geelong, Australia.

Sumner, J. and Danielson, E. (2007) Critical social theory as a means of analysis for caring in nursing. *International Journal for Human Caring*, 11(1), 30–7.

Walsh, E., Dilworth, S. and Freshwater, D. (2007) *Establishing Clinical Supervision in Prison Health Care Settings: Phase 3*. A report for Offender Health, Department of Health. Bournemouth University, Bournemouth.

Watson, R., Stimpson, A., Topping, A. and Porock, D. (2002) Clinical competence assessment in nursing: a systematic review of the literature. *Journal of Advanced Nursing*, 39(5), 421–31.

WHO (World Health Organization) (2000) *Munich Declaration: Nurses and midwives – a force for health*. World Health Organization, Copenhagen.

Chapter 10

Caring and reflection: the essence of nursing

Beverley J Taylor

Introduction

Nurses agree that care is central to nursing, making it an enormous task to grasp the ramifications of caring in nursing. The challenge of nursing scholarship has been taken up by caring theorists, who have developed theories and models to describe caring in the practice discipline of nursing. This chapter sets the context of caring, by reviewing foundational ideas within nursing scholarship, as a beginning place in which to locate commonalities that characterize and energize nurses' work. This chapter also suggests that caring and reflection are the essence of nursing, but that the identity and progress of both in the postmodern era depend on the vigilance of the nurses doing the work of nursing in practice, education, research and management.

Setting the context

Nursing scholarship has developed over time, attempting to define nursing in terms of the centrality of its practice and its associated concerns of research, education and management. Nursing literature has provided a medium through which to describe, debate and influence nursing and its positioning locally, nationally and globally, within the ever-widening realms of healthcare systems. These descriptions and debates have been immersed within the social, economic, cultural, political and historical contexts of their time. Through expositions in theses, books, journals and websites, nurses have engaged in, and continue to discuss, definitions of nursing, metaparadigm concepts, the nature and effects of nursing inherent in the nurse–patient relationship, caring and reflection. The complexity of the discussions and the parallel exponential growth in nursing scholarship reflects the enormity of nursing's influence within healthcare systems.

Definitions of nursing

Nurses are attempting to deal with the complexity of describing nursing, by paying attention to the metaparadigm domains of person, health, environment and nursing (Fawcett, 1989). This means that knowledge that can be claimed to be unique to nursing is concerned directly with any or all of the four domains that represent the scope of nursing. Given that the domains are broad, there are many interpretations of what constitutes nursing knowledge, by whom, how, and for what purposes. Therefore, nursing is defining itself continually through human health concerns inclusive of people in their environments, conveyed by ontological and epistemological means, as nurses come to know and understand their work and their relationships to themselves, other people and phenomena in nursing. Considered ontologically as lived experience, the nature of nursing is made manifest by locating and describing the embodied intricacies of everyday nurse–patient encounters.

Nursing occurs in social contexts, being influenced by multifactorial economic, cultural, political and historical determinants, which generate and potentially direct and distort intersubjective meanings. Nursing scholars set and consolidated the theoretical groundwork by expressing nursing from the interpretive, intersubjective viewpoints of its participants (Allen, 1985; Allen *et al.*, 1986; Banonis, 1989; Benner, 1984, 1985; Benner and Wrubel, 1989; Brown, 1986; Carper, 1978; Davis, 1973, 1978; Drew, 1986; Field and Morse, 1985; Forrest, 1989; Gulino, 1982; Hyde, 1977; McMahon and Pearson, 1991; McPherson, 1987; Mitchell, 1990; Parse, 1987; Paterson, 1971, 1978; Paterson and Zderad, 1976; Pearson, 1988, 1989; Taylor, 1992; Thompson, 1987; Watson, 1981, 1985), shifting away from nursing's focus on reductionist, biomedically oriented care (Frederick and Northam, 1938; Henderson, 1955; Nightingale, 1893; Orlando, 1961). Also, a turn towards critical viewpoints raises questions about the status quo and how nursing might redefine itself, in relation to poststructural and postmodern influences (Freshwater, 2002; Gadow, 1999; Gilbert, 2001; Kim, 1999; Watson, 1999).

Context is all-important in understanding and defining nursing. Contextually appropriate understandings and actions were described by Benner and Wrubel (1989: 412), who extended the general meaning of 'environment' as it was defined in nursing literature, to refer to 'situation,' which implies 'the relevant concerns, issues, information, constraints, and resources at a given span of time or place as experienced by particular persons.' Therefore, the way nurses and patients make sense of their situations will be 'in terms of their own personal concerns, background meanings, temporality, habitual, cultural bodies, emotions and reflective thoughts' (p. 82). It follows that the lived experience of nursing connects nurses and patients inextricably with the people and phenomena in their worlds, not only as people engaged in present dialog, but also as people embodying their past and anticipating their future.

Epistemological means of defining nursing have been connected to ontological perspectives (Abdellah *et al.*, 1960; Benner, 1984; Benner and Wrubel, 1989; Frederick and Northam, 1938; Henderson, 1955; King, 1971; Kinlein, 1977; Nightingale, 1893; Orem, 1959; Orlando, 1961; Paterson and Zderad, 1976; Peplau, 1952; Rogers, 1961; Roy, 1976; Travelbee, 1971; Wiedenbach, 1964) and to epistemological categories (Allen *et al.*, 1986; Carper, 1978; Chinn and Kramer, 1991; Parse, 1987).

Over time, nurses have used literature and discursive forums, such as professional conferences and seminars, to discuss and extend viewpoints of nursing. From Nightingale's (1893, in Seymer, 1954: 334–5) classic definition, that nursing puts 'us in the best possible conditions for Nature to restore or to preserve health – to prevent or to cure disease or injury,' to Frederick and Northam's (1938: 3) claim that 'nursing requires the application of scientific knowledge and nursing skills and affords the opportunities for constructive work in the care and relief of patients and their families,' and to Peplau's (1952: 16) description of nursing as 'a significant, therapeutic, interpersonal process,' nurses have attempted to identify the nature and effects of their work.

By asserting that nursing is about helping people to help themselves, Henderson (1955) ushered in an emphasis on self-care (Kinlein, 1977; Orem, 1959). Abdellah *et al.* (1960: 24) connected the notions of the knowledge base and the service of nursing and claimed that 'nursing is a service to individuals and to families; therefore, to society.' Orlando (1961), Rogers (1961) and Wiedenbach (1964) agreed about the supportive role of the nurse depicted by Nightingale, Henderson, Orem, Kinlein and Abdellah *et al.*, while Travelbee (1971: 7) agreed with Peplau, that nursing is 'an interpersonal process whereby the professional nurse practitioner assists an individual, family, or community to prevent or cope with the experience of illness and suffering and, if necessary, to find meaning in these experiences.'

King (1971) and Roy (1976) continued the theme of nursing as being supportive, influenced to some extent by the biomedical model of healthcare of the empirico-analytical tradition, yet they were careful to acknowledge the uniqueness of the nurse–patient relationship in the nursing exchange. Notwithstanding the difficulties in reaching definitional consensus, Erickson *et al.* (1983: 29) found commonalities in what nurses say collectively, with themes being evident of the mission of nursing to

> *assist persons; with their responses to health and illness states; with their self-care practices in relation to their health (with their coping and adapting); to achieve a state of (optimum) wellness by way of an interpersonal process.*

Nursing scholars have acknowledged the various ways of knowing, as evidenced by epistemological inquiries in philosophy and other human sciences (Allen *et al.*, 1986; Carper, 1978; Chinn and Kramer, 1991; Parse, 1987). Many of our contemporary discussions about nursing's epistemology take, as a starting point, Carper's (1978) four fundamental patterns of knowing in nursing: empirics, the science of nursing; esthetics, the art of nursing; the component of personal knowledge in nursing; and ethics, the moral component. Carper acknowledged the contribution of all the patterns of knowing in increasing nurses' awareness of the diversity and complexity of nursing knowledge, emphasizing that all forms of knowing have their place and none are mutually exclusive. Chinn and Kramer (1991) extended the acknowledgment of equal importance and mutual inclusiveness of Carper's patterns of knowing in nursing, by emphasizing the integrative aspects of knowing and describing the negative effects of 'patterns gone wild.'

Allen *et al.* (1986: 23) supported 'a pluralistic vision of research methodology' by describing three paradigms for generating knowledge within nursing: the empirico-analytical paradigm, Heideggerian phenomenology and critical social theory. These paradigms equate with Habermas' 'knowledge-constitutive interests' (Habermas, 1972), by falling into technical, practical and emancipatory categorizations respectively. The technical interests include empirico-analytical ways of knowing, practical interests include interpretive ways of knowing, and emancipatory interests include critical ways of knowing.

Parse (1987) reflected the simultaneity paradigm, unlike Peplau, Henderson, Hall, Orlando, Levine, Johnson, Roy, Orem and King, who reflected the totality paradigm, a natural or medical science approach to nursing. Parse (1987: 160) claimed that her work was a human science approach to nursing, viewing a person as 'a unitary being in continuous mutual interrelationship with the environment.' Regardless of the ways in which nursing scholars present their epistemological categorizations, there is continued agreement that alternatives to positivistic understandings exist (Freshwater, 2004; Freshwater and Avis, 2004; Freshwater and Stickley, 2004; Rolfe, 2001), and that nursing requires a mixture of epistemological approaches for finding meaning in nursing, to portray the relative complexity and diversity of knowledge in a practice discipline. Implicit in all of these definitions is the core business of nursing, as nurses care for, and give care to, people in need of their unique knowledge, skills and humanity.

Humanistic qualities in the nurse–patient relationship have been addressed in the literature, as authenticity, concern and presencing. From Jourard's (1971: 182) critique of the 'nurse's bedside manner,' as a facade to shield her or him from the vulnerability inherent in her or his own humanness, discussions of self-disclosure and authenticity have progressed, to allow possibilities for choices in nursing practice, as nurses decide courses of action in their day-to-day work (Benner, 1984; Benner and Wrubel, 1989; Parse, 1987).

Using the phenomenological concept of concern to describe person and interpersonal relationships as things that really matter, Benner and Wrubel (1989: 49) point out that although 'taking over' concern is necessary when patients are unable to cope by themselves, the 'giving back' solicitude 'is a form of advocacy and facilitation. It empowers the Other to be what he or she wants to be, and this is the ultimate goal in nursing care relationships.'

Presencing (Heidegger, 1962) describes the availability of the nurse to understand the patient, by a process of human relating. As Benner and Wrubel (1989: 13) explain, 'the ability to presence oneself, to be with the patient in a way that acknowledges your shared humanity, is the base of much of nursing as a caring practice.' This kind of nursing is akin to Campbell's (1985) 'skilled companionship,' that entails sharing freely and not imposing, thus allowing others to make their own life journey. He conceptualized nursing as involving a bodily presence, in sensing need and accommodating idiosyncrasies (sensitivity); in helping onwards to recovery or death (encouraging); in risking to be with, staying with the difficult point (being with); and in allowing the other to go on alone (limitation). Thus, Campbell (1985) saw nursing as a love-companionship relationship, involving sensitivity, being with, and allowing for limitation of the caring role, which fits with nursing's therapeutic nature and outcomes.

Nursing is both carative and curative (Benner and Wrubel, 1989; Kitson, 1984; Pearson, 1988), care is the essence of nursing (Leininger, 1985; Watson, 1985) as the most obvious and regularly described attribute of nursing, and nursing is a therapeutic relationship (McMahon and Pearson, 1991; Meutzel, 1988; Peplau, 1952; Pearson, 1988; Swaffield, 1988). All of these assertions are rich fields for reflective practice. We have recognized for some time that nurses become very skilled at doing things; 'doing for' is how they reflect their knowledge and skills and deliver nursing care. In a carative sense, 'doing for' is related to 'being with,' when nurses attend to the quality of the nurse–patient relationship, through which patients' goals are negotiated, set and accomplished (McPherson, 1987).

Essentially, nurses have been typified in nursing literature as dispensers of nursing care, within the authority of their professional roles. Nurses have been depicted as supporting the curative properties of Nature (Henderson, 1966; Nightingale, 1893), as facilitators of patients' stimulus-response mechanisms (Johnson, 1980; Orlando, 1961; Peplau, 1952; Roy, 1976) and as health professionals, who direct patients towards goal attainment (Abdellah *et al.*, 1960; Hall, 1964; King, 1971, 1981; Neuman, 1989; Orem, 1985; Wiedenbach, 1964). What had been less apparent in nursing practice and its supporting literature, especially until the advent of reflective practice discussions, were multiple strategies for nurses to transcend the confines of their role responsibilities and institutional expectations, to reflect critically on their work and revisit their own humanity.

Caring models and theories expressing the essence of nursing

Just as the task of describing nursing is enormous, so also is the task of grasping the ramifications of caring in nursing. Caring theorists have tackled this task and their work has been studied, researched and applied in nursing practice. Scholars develop theories and models to describe, organize or explain a phenomenon, or group of phenomena of a discipline, in a language appropriate to the discipline. Models and theories organize nursing knowledge in an orderly, coherent way, thus providing a 'map' of the knowledge of the discipline (Marriner-Tomey and Alligood, 2002; Rothrock and Smith, 2000; Smith, 2001; Walsh, 2000). Caring theories and models feature reflection implicitly and a selection of them are highlighted in this section, described briefly in chronological order, in relation to their foundational works (Peplau, 1952; Orem, 1959; Rogers, 1970; Levine, 1973; Paterson and Zderad, 1976; Roy, 1976; Leininger, 1978; Watson, 1979; Johnson, 1980; King, 1981; Neuman, 1982; Benner, 1984; Newman, 1986; Parse, 1987; Roach, 1987; Benner and Wrubel, 1989; Gadow, 1999; Boykin and Schoenhofer, 2001).

Hildegard Peplau is classified as a nursing theorist of historical significance (Marriner-Tomey, 2006), for her contribution of the Model of Psychodynamic Nursing (1952), contextualized within psychiatric nursing, which identifies four phases of the nurse–client interaction as orientation, identification, exploitation and resolution. Peplau described six nursing roles, specifically, stranger, resource person, teacher, leader, surrogate and counselor. She also discussed the psychobiological experiences of needs, frustrations, conflicts and anxieties, which evoke destructive or constructive responses.

Orem's (1959) model, the Self-Care Deficit Theory of Nursing, comprises three related theories: the theory of self-care, which describes and explains self-care; the theory of self-care deficit, which describes how clients need nursing; and the theory of nursing system, which describes and explains relationships necessary for nursing to take place. The theory of self-care deficit proposes that sometimes persons or their dependants have a greater need for self-care than they can fulfill, so an external source can assist, such as a nurse. The theory of nursing system links the nurse and the client through the provision of care, which can be wholly compensatory, in which the nurse performs all care for the client, partially compensatory, in which the nurse and client share the care, or supportive-educative, in which the nurse supports and educates the client.

Martha Rogers's Theory of Unitary Human Beings (1970) postulated that human beings are dynamic energy fields inseparable from their environmental energy fields. In Rogers's paradigm, the four major concepts are (1) energy fields, (2) a universe of open systems, (3) pattern and (4) pan-dimensionality. Rogers saw the fundamental unit of the living and the non-living as the energy field; therefore, a unitary human being is an energy field, not limited by time and space, with a unique pattern, the characteristics of which cannot be predicted from knowledge of the parts. The environmental energy field and the human energy field form open systems that exchange energy with each other, as they change constantly. Rogers described three principles of homeodynamics: the Principle of Helicy, or the continuous variety of human and environmental field patterns; the Principle of Integrality, or the continuous mutual human–environmental field interaction and processes, and the Principle of Resonancy, or change from lower to higher frequency of the wave patterns as the person develops and becomes more complex and moves towards pan-dimensionality.

Levine (1973) developed four Conservation Principles to provide a structure for teaching medical-surgical nursing. The four conservation principles are conservation of energy, of structural integrity, of personal integrity, and of social integrity. Levine's model views people as holistic beings, able to adapt and preserve their integrity with the external environment. If any of these principles is altered, the person's health status is changed. The nurse acts therapeutically to help the client conserve energy and maintain integrity or adapt to changes in energy or integrity. When further adaptation cannot occur, the nurse supports the individual and family while care is needed.

After years of experience in clinical practice and teaching, during which they identified the inability of positivistic science to address human phenomena in nursing, Paterson and Zderad (1976) formulated a humanistic nursing model. Based on phenomenological perspectives, they developed the construct of nursology, using phenomenological methods to pose questions and search for answers about nursing. Paterson and Zderad (1976: 19) conceptualized nursing as 'a lived act, a response to a human situation' and they described humanistic nursing as

> *the act of nursing, the intersubjective transactional relation, the dialogue experience, lived in concert between persons where comfort and nurturance prod mutual unfolding.* (Paterson and Zderad, 1976: 51)

The Roy (1976) Adaptation Model views the individual as a system adapting constantly, in response to stimuli from the external or internal environment. Stimuli can be classed as 'focal' immediate stimuli, 'contextual' contributing stimuli, or 'residual' background stimuli. Each person has levels of adaptation that contribute to the achievement of goals, such as survival or growth, and two mechanisms for responding to stimuli and controlling adaptation: the regulator or physiological mechanism, and the cognator or behavioral mechanism. Persons adapt in four modes. The physiological mode deals with physiological responses. The three psychosocial modes are the self-concept mode, which deals with psychic integrity; the role function mode, which deals with social roles; and the interdependence mode, which deals with interactions with other people.

Madeleine Leininger is 'the founder of transcultural nursing and a leader in transcultural nursing and human care theory' (McFarland, 2006: 472). She has been prolific in her contributions to nursing scholarship, from her earliest writings (Leininger, 1970, 1978) to the present day (Leininger and McFarland, 2006). McFarland (2006: 479) lists Leininger's major culture and care concepts and defines transcultural nursing as a

> *formal area of humanistic and scientific knowledge and practices focused on holistic culture care (caring) phenomena and competencies to assist individuals or groups to maintain or regain their health (or wellbeing) and to deal with disabilities, dying, or other human conditions in culturally congruent and beneficial ways.*

Jean Watson (1979) developed a model of ten carative factors for nurses to use in nursing encounters incorporating: formation of a humanistic-altruistic system of values; instillation of faith-hope; cultivation of sensitivity to self and to others; development of a helping-trusting relationship; promotion and acceptance of the expression of positive and negative feelings; systematic use of the scientific problem-solving method for decision making; promotion of interpersonal learning; provision for supportive, protective, corrective, mental, physical, sociocultural and spiritual environment; assistance with gratification of human needs; and allowance for existential phenomenological forces. Other important publications that have influenced nursing practice, education and research globally are *Nursing: Human Science and Human Care. A Theory of Nursing* (Watson, 1985) and *Postmodern Nursing and Beyond* (Watson, 1999).

Theories applying systems to human caring include Johnson's (1980) Behavioral Systems Model, which proposes seven behavioral subsystems that classify human behavior, including the biological subsystem and the achievement subsystem. In addition, King (1981) developed a Theory of Goal Attainment. King's model is a systems model that conceptualizes the person as an open system interacting with the environment, within a personal system as part of a group, and an interpersonal system, as part of a social system.

Neuman's (1982) systems model views the client's system as consisting of the basic structure or core, surrounded by layers of defenses. The basic structure or energy resources, comprising intrinsic human factors related to survival, such as genetic and ego structures, and regulation of body temperature, are surrounded immediately by the flexible lines of resistance, representing the body's resources that defend against stressors, for example, the immune system. Outside the flexible lines of resistance is the normal line of defense, which is a constant stability state for the individual who has adjusted to stressors. The outermost ring comprises the flexible lines of defense, which are shields against intrapersonal, interpersonal and extrapersonal stressors that may alter the stability of the system. The nurse acts, using prevention to intervene in the interaction of the client with stressors. Primary prevention occurs when a stressor is suspected or identified; secondary prevention occurs after symptoms from stress have occurred; and tertiary prevention occurs after the active treatment and leads back to primary prevention.

Benner (1984) was influenced by phenomenological perspectives of experience (Gadamer, 1975; Heidegger, 1962) and by notions of expert practice (Dreyfus and Dreyfus, 1980) to describe the knowledge embedded in expert nursing practice. Using paradigm cases around patient care issues, Benner (1984: 11) was able to define nursing practice at all levels of sophistication from novice to expert and conclude that

> *a wealth of untapped knowledge is embedded in the practices and the 'know-how' of expert nurse clinicians, but this knowledge will not expand or fully develop unless nurses systematically record what they learn from their own experience.*

Benner's Model of Skill Acquisition in Nursing (1984) used research to uncover the knowledge embedded in clinical practice. Benner has stated that 'the lack of charting of our practices and clinical observations deprives nursing theory of the uniqueness and richness of the knowledge embedded in clinical practice' (Benner, 1984: 2). This knowledge is central to the advancement of nursing practice and to the development of nursing science.

Margaret Newman's Model of Health as Expanding Consciousness (Newman, 1986) describes the core concepts of health, pattern, consciousness and movement-space-time. Health is disease and non-disease, which is a process of developing awareness as the person responds to the environment as 'the pattern of the whole' (Witucki Brown, 2006: 502). Pattern creates unity in diversity, as the person understands the meaning of all relationships. Consciousness includes cognitive and affective awareness and interconnectedness within oneself and all things, and movement-space-time are emerging patterns of consciousness.

Parse's (1987) model was developed using Rogers's model as a foundation, along with concepts from existential-phenomenological thought

(Lee *et al.*, 1994). Parse's model involves the notion that health is a lived experience, in which humans structure meaning multi-dimensionally, move towards greater diversity, and reach beyond the self.

Sister M. Simone Roach's work, *The Human Act of Caring: A Blueprint for the Health Professions*, asserts that 'caring is the human mode of being,' and that it is 'the most common, authentic criterion of humanness' (Roach, 1987: 2). She describes the five Cs of Compassion, Competence, Confidence, Conscience and Commitment and cautions us about the potential crisis of values in caring in insecure times.

Benner and Wrubel (1989: 7) focussed 'on the lived experiences of being healthy and being ill.' They claimed that the

> *best nursing practitioners understand the differences and relationships among health, illness and disease. This understanding leads nurses to seek the patient's story in formal and informal nursing histories, because they know that every illness has a story – plans that are threatened or thwarted, relationships are disturbed, and symptoms become laden with meaning depending on what else is happening in the person's life.* (Benner and Wrubel, 1989: 9)

Boykin and Schoenhofer (2001) describe 'nursing as caring: a model for transforming practice' and make this their book title. The major assumptions underlying their model are that: persons are caring by virtue of their humanness; persons are caring, moment to moment; persons are whole and complete in the moment; personhood is a process of living, grounded in caring; personhood is enhanced through participating in nurturing relationships with caring others; and nursing is both a discipline and a profession (Boykin and Schoenhofer, 2001: 1). They suggest that dialog and the retelling of nursing stories can provide nursing students with the 'opportunity to participate in a lived experience and to create new possibilities' (p. 45) and that search for the 'greater meaning of caring' can be enhanced by journaling (p. 46).

Sally Gadow (1999) suggests a postmodern turn in nursing ethics, away from the previous deontological, virtue and consequentialist categories of philosophical ethics to relational narrative. She explains the 'move from universalism to engagement is the turn from rational to relational ethics' (Gadow, cited in Kenney, 2003: 137), through valuing intersubjectivity and the voicing of layered meanings of 'an absurd ethics' within nursing care. Hence, relational narrative allows nurses and patients to co-create their own meanings within clinical settings, while not dismissing 'immersion and detachment as ethical approaches' (Gadow, in Kenney, 2003: 146).

This section overviewed the influential work of some nursing scholars who have contributed to the literature on human caring in nursing. These scholars agree that caring is central to nursing practice, and they present caring attitudes and behaviors in various ways to emphasize their particular concepts. The majority of the nurse scholars reviewed in this section paint a rosy picture of nursing, as respectful, skillful and knowledgable human-to-human care, in which only the best nursing attitudes, behaviors and outcomes are imagined. Although many scholars do not name reflection explicitly in their theories and models, these processes are implicit in human caring, as nurses continue to care thoughtfully for people, within caring contexts.

Reflexivity in caring

Returning to the first part of this chapter, we can see that nursing scholarship has developed over time, as nurses attempt to define nursing in terms of the centrality of its practice and its associated concerns of research, education and management. Even though these descriptions and debates have been immersed within the wider social, economic, cultural, political and historical contexts of their time, less attention has been paid in nursing literature to the constraining influences of these contexts and authors have remained relatively silent on the politics of interpersonal relationships and of healthcare systems.

Definitions of nursing have addressed the metaparadigm domains of person, health, environment and nursing in mainly humanistic, interpretive accounts of lived experience and the potential of the ways of knowing in nurse–patient encounters. Theories and models of nursing have also embraced the inherent positive values of humanness, emphasizing the therapeutic nature of undistorted human relationships, within settings that are assumed to work for the 'good of the patient.' Even though these definitions, models and theories have inherent worth and are positive in their hopefulness for the highest good of the nurse–patient relationship, they tend to overlook or temporarily ignore the less-than-ideal characteristics of care and caring that lie within and between human relationships and healthcare settings and organizations. To some extent, these areas are being highlighted by the turn in nursing literature towards critical and postmodern descriptions of the human condition and research approaches (see Chapter 2), but much has yet to be done to identify and deal with less-than-caring behaviors in toxic healthcare settings, and the politics of nursing care generally, in the wider realm of budget-constrained healthcare systems.

While writers agree generally that caring is central to nursing practice, and nursing has made a paradigm shift to qualitative research epistemologies, there is also a growing debate about the politics of healthcare and how caring behaviors can be assessed in the Western world, which is demanding a return to quantitative research methods, as the best indication of evidence-based practice. Power is inherent in human relationships and the politics of care is 'alive and well' in nursing practice, just as it is in any situation in which people share, and to various extents, compete for, common interests and goals. Knowledge is power also, and it can be used intentionally as a political instrument, or have its effect as reified dogma, thereby silencing critique and stultifying change strategies. Therefore, in the light of the increasing complexity in healthcare politics and the need for nursing to re-evaluate itself within those systems constantly, caring must include reflexivity, as a means of improving oneself and the practice discipline of nursing, while maintaining vigilance in caring.

Views that question and extend foundational thinking in nursing are being expressed in professional refereed journal articles which are providing the medium for debate. For example, Heath (1998a) discussed reflection and patterns of knowing, extending Carper's (1978) typology to include two more categories: unknowing and sociopolitical knowing. Acknowledging Munhall's (1993) idea of unknowing as an art, Heath (1998a: 1057) contends that 'unknowing is related to all patterns' of knowing, and its value lies in alertness and remaining open to what is not known and what might emerge in any situation. Sociopolitical knowing highlights constraints and competing forces in healthcare settings. Heath (1998a) suggested that nurses might have difficulty applying knowledge forms to their practice and see it as an academic exercise, not immediately urgent in their busy work settings. Hence, the extension of knowledge into the unknown and sociopolitical categories creates room for movement in practice that captures clinical concerns. The inclusion of these types of knowing allows for the possibilities of uncertainty and distorting factors in caring contexts and encourages nurses to establish a culture of critique in their workplaces.

In relation to care, Cloyes (2002: 203) examines the 'tensions between care feminism and agonistic feminism . . . in order to explore the potential of theorizing both care and nursing in political terms.' She traces the progress of the caring literature and concludes that, with the exception of care ethics and feminist thought, the idea of care as central to nursing theory and practice has largely gone unchallenged. She argues for shifting the

conversation about care, care theory and care ethics away from approaches that either uncritically valorize care or frame constructs of care within dichotomizing and ultimately reifying terms of either 'care versus justice' or 'contextualized versus uncontextualized frameworks'. (Cloyes, 2002: 204)

Cloyes (2002: 209) traces the evolution of critical accounts of care in nursing and care ethics and questions whether 'we can bridge the discourses of care ethics and politics without resorting to either masculinist or maternalist models.' Cloyes (2002: 210) offers the possibility of agonistic feminism, which assumes that care is 'ideological and that "care" is itself implicated in power relations,' therefore, agonistic feminists 'frame their critique as political intervention.' Identifying and transforming the ramifications of these political assumptions about care requires a sustained and systematic commitment to reflective practice strategies.

Alongside the critiques of care that shift nursing discourses beyond interpretive accounts to critical and postmodern representations, there is a powerful counter-pull back towards measuring caring behaviors so that they count as credible knowledge in evidence-based practice. Just as power and the politics of care is 'alive and well' in nursing practice, so also is the dominant discourse of the biomedical model, expressed in measurable terms in the levels of evidence for practice, gained primarily through quantitative research methods. This counter-pull to the epistemological superiority of quantitative research is discussed elsewhere in this book (see Chapter 2).

Consequently, some nurse researchers are attempting to measure care quantitatively, for example: by testing a care model using a correlation survey design (Suhonen *et al.*, 2004); psychometric testing on the Nurse–Patient Interactions Scale to assess nurse–patient interactions from a caring perspective (Cossette *et al.*, 2005); measuring peer caring behaviors of nursing students (Kou *et al.*, 2007); measuring perceptions of caring among student nurses using a caring dimensions inventory (Watson *et al.*, 2001); and measuring nurse caring behaviors using a Care-Q instrument (Greenhalgh *et al.*, 1998).

The underlying assumptions in using these objective methods are that care is observable in nursing practice and education and that it can be measured by empirico-analytical means. While this may be so to some extent, the levels of evidence in evidence-based practice, globally, dismiss intersubjective understandings of human health and pay little respect also to critiques of power and knowledge inherent in poststructural and postmodern epistemologies. This puts nursing in a difficult place; having made a move to broader views of the human experience of health and illness, nursing now finds itself needing to choose between a commitment to nursing as intersubjective, contextualized relationships, or nursing as objectified, cause-and-effect relationships, or to shift somewhere in between according to the expediencies of healthcare and research resources and disciplinary credibility.

Increasingly, authors are agreeing that care and caring are difficult concepts (Bassett, 2002; Eklund-Myrskog, 2000; McCance *et al.*, 1997), that they are gendered concepts (Cloyes, 2002; Poole and Isaacs, 1997) and that nursing needs to provide multiple forms of evidence for their claims of the beneficial effects of care (Pearson, 2002; Rolfe, 1997; Watson and Foster, 2003). This being so, nursing needs to build on its rich heritage of scholarship, inherent in practice, education, research and management, to move forward with multiple epistemologies that embrace change, difference and diversity. Reflective practice is inclusive and respectful of all the epistemologies embraced thus far in nursing theory and practice, while offering technical, practical and emancipatory possibilities for examining and extending understandings of self and others, within the complexities of caring, in practice settings rife with social, economic, cultural, political and historical influences and constraints.

Maintaining vigilance in caring through reflective practice

While it may be argued convincingly that caring and reflection are the essence of nursing, the identity and progress of both paradigms depends on the vigilance of the nurses doing the daily work of nursing in practice, education, research and management, and their ability to influence levels of government and peak health organizations, the representatives of which set health initiatives and policies and allocate resources accordingly. The complexity of nursing practice requires strategies for maintaining vigilance in planning, giving and evaluating nursing care, and this vigilance needs to be just as robust and constant in the associated areas of nursing research, education and management.

Nursing literature has described and debated the value of thinking processes that enhance the formation of effective knowledge, skills and humanity in nursing practice. For example, authors agree that conceptual acuity in problem solving (Anderson, 1996; Eunson, 2005; Liberman *et al.*, 2001) and critical thinking (Bandman and Bandman, 1995; Kenney, 2003; van Hooft *et al.*, 1995; Wilkinson, 1996) is essential in ensuring safe and effective communication, decision making, conflict resolution and care delivery in nursing practice. While guidance is offered to some extent in how to achieve the levels of conceptual acuity required for higher-order thinking inherent in effective communication, decision making, conflict resolution and care delivery, there is no guide book written, nor could it ever be compiled, to help nurses to get everything correct, always, and on time, in the immediacy of practice. This means that there are always possibilities for things to go wrong, or to be less than ideal, for nurses working in any field of nursing, but especially in practice, where clinical thinking has real and rapid consequences. While nurses cannot stop 'bad things' happening, they need to be vigilant constantly to the possibility of things going wrong, to prevent them if possible, and to adjust the processes and systems of care, so that they are less likely to happen again. This vigilance is enhanced by reflection-in and on-action, which is discussed throughout this book.

Reflective practice is a system of thinking that can assist nurses in maintaining vigilance in caring. It does not oppose, or compete with, successful systems of thought and thinking already adopted in nursing; rather it seeks to organize various modes of thinking into a collective of methods and processes that can work together to enhance the reflective abilities of nurses in their workplaces, wherever they might be.

Much of the focus on reflective practice is on the work of nursing, as practiced in clinical caring contexts (Freshwater, 1998, 2002; Glaze, 1999; Heath, 1998a, b; Johns, 2000, 2003; Taylor, 2004, 2006; Wilkin, 2002). For example, Freshwater (1998) provided a meta-analysis of reflection and caring using the analogy of the acorn becoming an oak tree. To emphasize the role of reflection in nurses' personal and professional development, Freshwater used an awakening and growth analogy, and suggested that 'reflective practice helps us to explore what is just beyond the line of vision, it encourages not to stare straight ahead, but to turn around' (Freshwater, 1998: 16).

Heath (1998b) described the experiences of clinicians in keeping reflective journals of their practice. Based on the experiences of continuing education students, Heath was able to offer practical guidance in writing reflectively, to gain deeper levels of reflective awareness in learning, practice implications, relevance and applicability, conclusions and wider context constraints and action.

Glaze (1999: 30) described reflection, clinical judgment and staff development 'to encourage perioperative nurses to reflect on their practice.' She used exemplars of expert practice 'to illustrate how knowledge is used and developed in the practice setting.' The outcomes of reflection include practical advice and insights into how perioperative nurses may improve their practice.

Johns (2000: 199) reflected on his own practice of 'working with Alice,' which assisted him to draw 'out key issues of practice and reflection that enabled [him] to gain insight and apply to future practice within a reflexive learning spiral.' Through clear and thoughtful writing, Johns describes Alice's appearance, their conversation, and his part in it, reflecting-in-action on his words and their effect on Alice. Through this encounter he was able to raise reflective questions for himself and other nurses in the unit in relation to Alice's care.

Wilkin (2002) explored expert practice through reflection, by focussing on a clinical experience of caring for a 12-year-old boy diagnosed with brain death, and her experience of remaining on duty in the unit to facilitate the parent's wishes concerning his care. Wilkin (2002: 88) used 'the unusual experience . . . to enable self-criticism and expansion of personal knowledge,' in order to explore the complexity of expert practice and to facilitate holistic care.

Taylor's writing centers on reflection in nursing practice, for example, in giving advice for technical, practical and emancipatory reflection for practicing holistically (Taylor, 2004), and by providing a model of reflection for use in nursing and midwifery practice settings (Taylor, 2006).

Reflective practice has also been applied effectively in nurse education (Anderson and Branch, 2000; Clegg, 2000; Cruickshank, 1996; Freshwater, 1999; Kenney, 2003; Kim, 1999; Lian, 2001; Platzer *et al.*, 2000a, b). For example, Kim (1999: 1205) described 'a method of inquiry which uses nurses' situated, individual instances of nursing practice as the basis for developing knowledge for nursing and improving practice.' Using ideas from action science, critical philosophy and reflective practice, she described a critical reflective inquiry method and process that allows nurses to raise their awareness of their work constraints to free themselves towards more informed and liberating insights about their work.

Freshwater (1999: 28) undertook a research project to explore 'the lived experience of student nurses during a three year Diploma of Nursing program.' The students and tutor (researcher) examined 'how their own personal stories interfaced with those of the patient.' The students and tutor kept a reflective journal pertaining to their experiences of moving from perceived levels of novice to expert nurse. The project demonstrated how self-awareness through reflective practice and other strategies, such as clinical supervision and experiential learning, enhance personal and professional development in the clinical area.

Platzer *et al.* (2000b: 689) set up reflective practice groups in a post-registration nursing course 'to enable students to reflect on and learn from their experience.' The learning was evaluated through in-depth interviews and although students identified barriers to their learning, 'some students made significant developments in their critical thinking ability and underwent perspective transformations that led to changes in attitudes and behaviours.'

Anderson and Branch (2000: 1) endorsed the use of storytelling to promote critical reflection in Registered Nurse students, as 'a mechanism for one to talk about past actions as well as the results to these actions,' for giving voice to experiences, and 'revisiting the past for the purpose of shaping the future.' She concluded that 'adult educators can benefit tremendously from further research' that involves creative methodologies, such as storytelling and reflection.

Many more examples of the effectiveness of reflective practice in all areas of nursing are located within this book. These examples serve to make the point that reflective practice is effective and that the complexity of nursing requires nurses to use all of the available systems of thinking within their grasp to maintain their vigilance in upholding the mission of nursing as a humanitarian service to those people in need of our knowledge, skills and humanity. Nurses must keep up with modes of thinking and creative practices if they are to thrive in the postmodern era, and this process begins with oneself and moves outwards towards others.

Freshwater (2002: 225) asserts that self-awareness 'is deemed to be central to the process of successful reflection, with the "self" being the main instrument of both the practice and guidance of reflection.' In a postmodern description of the process of guided reflection, Freshwater (2002: 225) explores 'some of the reflections that took place in the pauses between the lines of the text in the act of looking up from the reading' in order to 'bring light to bear in certain elements of the text, whilst recognizing that this casts a shadow on other aspects of the dialog.' In this writing, Freshwater (2002) captures deftly the postmodern puzzle of partialities, gaps, silences and shifts in meaning, while resting on the assurance that an exploration of self is a reflective exercise that offers some insights into local truths.

Summary

This chapter overviewed the influential work of some nursing scholars, who have contributed to the discourse on human caring in nursing with theories and models. These scholars agree that caring is central to nursing practice, and they present caring attitudes and behaviors in their particular concepts. The majority of the nurse scholars reviewed in this chapter represent nursing as respectful, skillful and knowledgable human-to-human care, in which only the best nursing attitudes, behaviors and outcomes are imagined. Although many scholars do not name reflection explicitly in their caring theories and models, these processes are implicit in human caring, as nurses continue to care thoughtfully for people, within caring contexts.

Even though descriptions of and debates about nursing have occurred within the wider social, economic, cultural, political and historical contexts of their time, relatively little attention has been paid in nursing literature to the constraining influences of these healthcare contexts and authors have remained relatively silent on the politics of interpersonal relationships within healthcare systems. Humanistic accounts of lived experience and the potential of the ways of knowing in nurse–patient encounters have embraced the inherent positive values of humanness, emphasizing the therapeutic nature of undistorted human relationships, within relatively ideal work settings. Even though these definitions, models and theories are noteworthy for their hopefulness for the highest good of the nurse–patient relationship, they tend to miss the less-than-ideal characteristics of care and caring, within and between human relationships, healthcare settings and organizations. Nursing does not always happen in positive relationships and settings, nor does it always have ideal outcomes, even with the best of intentions, so nursing needs established, systematic reflective processes to allow nurses to reflect critically on every aspect of their work procedures and policies, interpersonal relationships, and issues of power.

Given the growing debate in nursing about the politics of healthcare and how caring behaviors can be assessed in the Western world, as the best indication of evidence-based practice, together with the challenges of multiple epistemologies in the 21st century, nursing needs reflective processes that are effective in navigating the maze of nursing and healthcare. This chapter suggested that we can gain some assurance from caring and reflection as the combined essence of nursing, but we must remain vigilant to maintain their identity and progress in nursing in practice, education, research and management.

References

Abdellah, F.G., Beland, I.L., Martin, A. and Matheney, R.V. (1960) *Patient-Centered Approaches to Nursing*. Macmillan, New York.

Allen, D. (1985) Nursing research and social control: alternative models of nursing that emphasize understanding and emancipation. *Image*, 17(2), 58–64.

Allen, D., Benner, P. and Diekelmann, N.L. (1986) Three paradigms for nursing research: methodological implications, in Chinn, P.L. (ed.) *Nursing Research Methodology: Issues and Implementation*. Aspen, Rockville, MD.

Anderson, J.M. (ed.) (1996) *Thinking Management: Contemporary Approaches for Nurse Managers*. Ausmed Publications, Melbourne.

Anderson, M. and Branch, M. (2000) Storytelling: a tool to promote critical reflection in the RN student. *Minority Nurse Newsletter*, 71, 1–2.

Bandman, E.L. and Bandman, B. (1995) *Critical Thinking in Nursing*, 2nd edn. Appleton & Lange, Norwalk, CT.

Banonis, B.C. (1989) The lived experience of recovering from addiction: a phenomenological study. *Nursing Science Quarterly*, 2, 37–43.

Bassett, C. (2002) Nurses' perceptions of care and caring, *International Journal of Nursing Practice*, 8, 8–15.

Benner, P. (1984) *From Novice to Expert: Uncovering the Knowledge Embedded in Clinical Practice*. Addison-Wesley, Menlo Park, CA.

Benner, P. (1985) Quality of life: a phenomenological perspective on explanation prediction and understanding in nursing science. *Advances in Nursing Science*, 8(1), 1–14.

Benner, P. and Wrubel, J. (1989) *The Primacy of Caring: Stress and Coping in Health and Illness*. Addison-Wesley, Menlo Park, CA.

Boykin, A. and Schoenhofer, S.A. (2001) *Nursing as Caring: A Model for Transforming Practice*. National League for Nursing, New York.

Brown, L. (1986) The experience of care: patient perspectives. *Topics in Clinical Nursing*, 8(2), 56–62.

Campbell, A.V. (1985) *Paid to Care? The Limits of Professionalism in Pastoral Care*. SPCK/Anchor Press, London.

Carper, B. (1978) Fundamental ways of knowing in nursing. *Advances in Nursing Science*, 1(1), 13–23.

Chinn, P.L. and Kramer, M.K. (1991) *Theory and Nursing: A Systematic Approach*, 3rd edn. Mosby, St Louis, MO.

Clegg, S. (2000) Knowing through reflective practice in higher education. *Education Action Research*, 8(3), 451–69.

Cloyes, K.G. (2002) Agonizing care: care ethics, agonistic feminism and a political theory of care. *Nursing Inquiry*, 9(3), 203–14.

Cossette, S., Cara, C., Ricard, N. and Pepin, J. (2005) Assessing nurse–patient interactions from a caring perspective: Report of the development and preliminary psychometric testing of the Caring Nurse–Patient Interactions Scale. *International Journal of Nursing Studies*, 42, 673–86.

Cruickshank, D. (1996) The 'art' of reflection: using drawing to uncover knowledge development in student nurses. *Nurse Education Today*, 16(2), 127–30.

Davis, A. (1973) The Phenomenological Approach in Nursing Research, in Garrison, E. (ed.) *Doctoral Preparation for Nurses*. University of California, San Francisco.

Davis, A. (1978) The phenomenological approach in nursing research, in Chaska, N. (ed.) *The Nursing Profession: Views Through the Mist*. McGraw-Hill, New York.

Drew, N. (1986) Exclusion and confirmation: a phenomenology of patients' experiences with caregivers. *IMAGE: Journal of Nursing Scholarship*, 18(2), 39–43.

Dreyfus, S.E. and Dreyfus, H.L. (1980) *A five-stage model of mental activities involved in directed skill acquisition*. Unpublished report supported by the Air Force Office of Scientific Research, University of California, Berkeley, CA.

Eklund-Myrskog, D.G. (2000) Student nurses' understanding of caring science. *Nurse Education Today*, 20, 164–70.

Erickson, H.C., Tomlin, M. and Swain, M.A. (1983) *Modeling and Remodeling: A Theory and Paradigm for Nursing*. Prentice-Hall, Englewood Cliffs, NJ.

Eunson, B. (2005) *Conflict Management: Communicating in the 21st Century*. John Wiley & Sons, Brisbane, Australia.

Fawcett, J. (1989) *Analysis and Evaluation of Conceptual Models of Nursing*, 2nd edn. F.A. Davis, Philadelphia, PA.

Field, P. and Morse, J. (1985) *Nursing Research: The Application of Qualitative Approaches*. Croom Helm, London.

Forrest, D. (1989) The experience of caring. *Journal of Advanced Nursing*, 14, 815–23.

Frederick, H. and Northam, E. (1938) *A Textbook of Nursing Practice*. Macmillan, New York.

Freshwater, D. (1998) From acorn to oak tree: a neoplatonic perspective of reflection and caring. *Australian Journal of Holistic Nursing*, 5(2), 14–19.

Freshwater, D. (1999) Clinical supervision, reflective practice and guided discovery: clinical supervision. *British Journal of Nursing*, 8(20), 1383–9.

Freshwater, D. (2002) Guided reflection in the context of post-modern practice, in Johns, C. (ed.) *Guided Reflection: Advancing Practice*. Blackwell Science, Oxford.

Freshwater, D. (2004) Reflection: a tool for developing clinical leadership. *Reflections on Nursing Leadership*, 2nd quarter, 20–6.

Freshwater, D. and Avis, M. (2004) Analysing interpretation and reinterpreting analysis: exploring the logic of critical reflection. *Nursing Philosophy*, 5, 4–11.

Freshwater, D. and Stickley, T. (2004) The heart of the art: emotional intelligence in nurse education. *Nursing Inquiry*, 11(2), 91–8.

Gadamer, H.-G. (1975) *Truth and Method*. Barden, G. and Cumming, J. (eds and trans). Seabury Press, New York.

Gadow, S. (1999) Relational narrative: the postmodern turn in nursing ethics, in Kenney, J.W. *Philosophical and Theoretical Perspectives for Advanced Nursing Practice*, 3rd edn. Jones and Bartlett, Boston, pp. 137–47.

Gilbert, T. (2001) Reflective practice and supervision: meticulous rituals of the confessional. *Journal of Advanced Nursing*, 36(2), 199–205.

Glaze, J. (1999) Reflection, clinical judgment and staff development. *British Journal of Theatre Nursing*, 9(1), 30–4.

Greenhalgh, J., Vanhanen, L. and Kyngas, H. (1998) Nurse caring behaviours. *Journal of Advanced Nursing*, 27, 927–32.

Gulino, C.K. (1982) Entering the mysterious dimensions of others: an existential approach to nursing care. *Nursing Outlook*, 30(6), 352–7.

Habermas, J. (1972) *Knowledge and Human Interests*. Heinemann, London.

Hall, L.E. (1964) Nursing: what is it? *The Canadian Nurse*, 60(2), 150–4.

Heath, H. (1998a) Reflection and patterns of knowing in nursing. *Journal of Advanced Nursing*, 27(5), 1054–9.

Heath, H. (1998b) Keeping a reflective practice diary: a practical guide. *Nurse Education Today*, 18(7), 592–8.

Heidegger, M. (1962) *Being and Time*. Macquarrie, J. and Robinson, E. (trans). Harper & Row, New York.

Henderson, V. (1955) *Textbook of Principles and Practice of Nursing*. Macmillan, New York.

Henderson, V. (1966) *The Nature of Nursing*. Macmillan, New York.

Hyde, A. (1977) The phenomenon of caring. Part VI. *American Nurses' Foundation*, 12(1), 2.

Johns, C. (2000) Working with Alice: a reflection. *Complementary Therapies in Nursing and Midwifery*, 6, 199–303.

Johns, C. (2003) Easing into the light. *International Journal for Human Caring*, 7(1), 49–55.

Johnson, D.E. (1980) The behavioural system for nursing, in Riehl, J.P. and Roy, C. (eds) *Conceptual Models for Nursing Practice*, 2nd edn. Appleton-Century-Crofts, New York.

Jourard, S.M. (1971) *The Transparent Self*. Van Nostrand Reinhold, New York.

Kenney, L.J. (2003) Using Edward de Bono's six hats game to aid critical thinking and reflection in palliative care. *International Journal of Palliative Nursing*, 9(3), 105–12.

Kim, H.S. (1999) Critical reflective inquiry for knowledge development in nursing practice. *Journal of Advanced Nursing*, 29(5), 1205–12.

King, I.M. (1971) *Toward a Theory for Nursing: General Concepts of Human Behaviour*. John Wiley, New York.

King, I.M. (1981) *A Theory for Nursing: Systems Concepts Process*. John Wiley, New York.

Kinlein, M.L. (1977) *Independent Nursing Practice with Clients*. Lippincott, Philadelphia, PA.

Kitson, A.L. (1984) Steps towards the identification and development of nursing therapeutic functions in the care of hospitalised elderly. Unpublished PhD thesis, University of Ulster, Coleraine.

Kou, C.-L., Turton, M.A., Lee-Hsieh, J., Tseng, H.-F. and Hsu, C.-L. (2007) Measuring peer caring behaviours of nursing students: scale development. *International Journal of Nursing Studies*, 44, 105–14.

Lee, R., Schumacher, L. and Twigg, P. (1994) Rosemarie Rizzo Parse: man-living-health, in Marriner-Tomey, A. (ed.) *Nursing Theorists and Their Work*, 3rd edn. C.V. Mosby, St Louis, MO.

Leininger, M.M. (1970) *Nursing and Anthropology: Two Worlds to Blend*. John Wiley & Sons, New York.

Leininger, M.M. (1978) *Transcultural Nursing: Concepts, Theories and Practices*. John Wiley & Sons, New York.

Leininger, M. (1985) *Qualitative Research Methods in Nursing*. Grune & Stratton, New York.

Leininger, M.M. and McFarland, M.R. (2006) *Culture Care Diversity and Universality: A Worldwide Nursing Theory*, 2nd edn. Jones & Bartlett, Boston, MA.

Levine, M.E. (1973) *Introduction to Clinical Nursing*, 2nd edn. F.A. Davis, Philadelphia, PA.

Lian, J.X. (2001) Reflective practice: a critical incident. *Contemporary Nurse*, 3–4, 217–21.

Liberman, R.P., Hilty, D.M., Drake, R.E. and Tsang, H.W.H. (2001) Requirements for multidisciplinary teamwork in psychiatric rehabilitation. *Psychiatric Services*, 52(10), 1331–42.

McCance, T.V., McKenna, H.P. and Boore, J.R.P. (1997) Caring: dealing with a difficult concept. *International Journal of Nursing Studies*, 34(4), 241–8.

McFarland, M. (2006) Culture care theory of diversity and universality, in Marriner-Tomey, A. and Alligood, M.R. (eds) *Nursing Theorists and Their Work*, 6th edn. Mosby, St Louis, MO, 472–96.

McMahon, R. and Pearson, A. (eds) (1991) *Nursing as Therapy*. Chapman & Hall, London.

McPherson, P. (1987) The quality of being expressed as doing. *Australian Journal of Advanced Nursing*, 5(1), 38–42.

Marriner-Tomey, A. (2006) Nursing theorists of historical significance, in Marriner-Tomey, A. and Alligood, M.R. (eds) *Nursing Theorists and Their Work*, 6th edn. Mosby, St Louis, MO.

Marriner-Tomey, A. and Alligood, M.R. (eds) (2002) *Nursing Theorists and Their Work*, 5th edn. Mosby, St Louis, MO.

Meutzel, P.A. (1988) Therapeutic nursing, in Pearson, A. (ed.) *Primary Nursing*. Croom Helm, London.

Munhall, P. (1993) 'Unknowing': towards another pattern of knowing in nursing. *Nursing Outlook*, 41(3), 125–8.

Neuman, B.M. (1982) *The Neuman Systems Model: An Application to Nursing Education and Practice*. Appleton-Century-Crofts, Norwalk, CT.

Neuman, B. (1989) *The Neuman Systems Model*. Appleton & Lange, Norwalk, CT.

Newman, M. (1986) *Health as Expanding Consciousness*. National League for Nursing, New York.

Nightingale, F. (1893) *Selected Writings of Florence Nightingale*, compiled by Seymer, L. (1954). Macmillan, New York.

Orem, D. (1959) *Guides for Developing Curricula for the Education of Practical Nurses*. Government Printing Office, Washington, DC.

Orem, D.E. (1985) *Nursing: Concepts of Practice*, 3rd edn. McGraw-Hill, New York.

Orlando, I.J. (1961) *The Dynamic Nurse–Patient Relationship*. Putnam, New York.

Parse, R.R. (1987) *Nursing Science: Major Paradigms Theories and Critiques*. W.B. Saunders, Philadelphia, PA.

Paterson, J. and Zderad, L. (1976) *Humanistic Nursing*. Wiley, New York.

Pearson, A. (ed.) (1988) *Primary Nursing*. Croom Helm, London.

Pearson, A. (2002) Nursing takes the lead: redefining what counts as evidence in Australian health care. *Reflections on Nursing Leadership*, 4th quarter, 18–21.

Peplau, H.E. (1952) *Interpersonal Relations in Nursing*. Putnam, New York.

Platzer, H., Blake, D. and Ashford, D. (2000a) Barriers to learning from reflection: a study of the use of groupwork with post-registration nurses. *Journal of Advanced Nursing*, 31(5), 1001–8.

Platzer, H., Blake, D. and Ashford, D. (2000b) An evaluation of process and outcomes from learning through reflective practice groups on a post-registration nursing course. *Journal of Advanced Nursing*, 31(3), 689–95.

Poole, M. and Isaacs, D. (1997) Caring: a gendered concept. *Women's Studies International Forum*, 20(4), 529–36.

Roach, M.S. (1987) *The Human Act of Caring: A Blueprint for the Health Professions*. Canadian Hospital Association, Ottawa, Canada.

Rogers, M. (1961) *Educational Revolution in Nursing*. Macmillan, New York.

Rogers, M.E. (1970) *The Theoretical Basis of Nursing*. F.A. Davis, Philadelphia, PA.

Rolfe, G. (1997) Beyond expertise: theory, practice and the reflexive practitioner. *Journal of Clinical Nursing*, 6, 93–7.

Rolfe, G. (2001) Reflective practice: Where now? *Nurse Education in Practice*, 2, 21–9.

Rothrock, J. and Smith, D. (2000) Selecting the perioperative patient focused model. *AORN Journal*, 71(5), 1030–2, 1034, 1036–7.

Roy, C. (1976) *Introduction to Nursing: An Adaptation Model*. Prentice-Hall, Englewood Cliffs, NJ.

Smith, M. (2001) Analysis and evaluation of contemporary nursing knowledge: nursing models and theories. *Nursing and Health Care Perspectives*, 22(2), 92–3.

Suhonen, R., Valimaki, M., Leino-Kilpi, H. and Katajisto, J. (2004) Testing the individualized care model. *Scandinavian Journal of Caring Science*, 18, 27–36.

Swaffield, L. (1988) Communication: tuned in. *Nursing Times*, 84(23), 28–31.

Taylor, B.J. (2004) Technical, practical and emancipatory reflection for practising holistically. *Journal of Holistic Nursing*, 22(1), 73–84.

Taylor, B.J. (2006) *Reflective Practice: A Guide for Nurses and Midwives*, 2nd edn. Open University Press, Milton Keynes, UK.

Travelbee, J. (1971) *Interpersonal Aspects of Nursing*. F.A. Davis, Philadelphia, PA.

van Hooft, S., Gillam, L. and Byrnes, M. (1995) *Facts and Values: An Introduction to Critical Thinking for Nurses*. Maclennan & Petty, Sydney.

Walsh, M. (2000) Chaos, complexity and nursing. *Nursing Standard*, 14(32), 39–42.

Watson, J. (1979) *Nursing: The Philosophy and Science of Caring*. Little & Brown, Boston, MA.

Watson, J. (1981) Nursing's scientific quest. *Nursing Outlook*, 29(7), 413–16.

Watson, J. (1985) *Nursing: Human Science and Human Care. A Theory of Nursing*. Appleton-Century-Crofts, Norwalk, CT.

Watson, J. (1999) *Postmodern Nursing and Beyond*. Churchill-Livingstone, London.

Watson, J. and Foster, R. (2003) The Attending Nurse Caring Model: Integrating theory, evidence and advanced caring-healing therapeutics for transforming professional practice. *Journal of Clinical Nursing*, 12, 360–5.

Watson, R., Deary, I.J. and Hoogbruin, A.L. (2001) A 35-item version of the caring dimensions inventory (CDI-35): multivariate analysis and application to a longitudinal study involving student nurses. *International Journal of Nursing Studies*, 38, 511–21.

Wiedenbach, E. (1964) *Clinical Nursing: A Helping Art*. Springer Publishing, New York.

Wilkin, K. (2002) Exploring expert practice through reflection. *Nursing in Critical Care*, 7(2), 88–93.

Wilkinson, J.M. (1996) *Nursing Process: A Critical Thinking Approach*. Addison-Wesley, Menlo Park, CA.

Witucki Brown, J. (2006) Newman's theory of health as expanding consciousness in nursing practice, in Alligood, M.R. and Marriner-Tomey, A. (eds) *Nursing Theory: Utilization and Application*, 3rd edn. Mosby, St Louis, MO, 461–83.

Chapter 11

Reflective narratives: developing a career pathway

Dawn Freshwater and Philip Esterhuizen

Introduction

Nurse education has been and, it could be argued, continues, rather like healthcare, to be in a constant metamorphosis of evolution and change. The direction that nurse education should take is a topic that has been surrounded by controversy, fueled by the prevailing social, economic and political attitudes. Radical change brought about by the transfer of nurse education in institutes of higher education came about at the same time as economic stringency for healthcare in general. Both healthcare and nurse education continues in this vein today.

Nearly two decades ago Powell (1989) noted that the lack of available monies would not only impact nurse education, particularly continuing education for qualified nurses, but would also influence the future of nurse education, given the simultaneous drive for advanced nursing practice. This is problematic for there is little doubt that nurse education is an important area for policy makers, researchers and practitioners, given that its development can be viewed as a means to enhance patient care through nursing care and the nursing profession (Johns, 1995). Powell (1989) recommended that nurse education should acquire a deeper and higher understanding of nursing and its contributing disciplines. However, she also commented that this deeper understanding needed to come from practice and applied knowledge, suggesting reflective practice as a way forward. Many writers (1993) are in accord with this view, concurring that practice experience is central to nurse education.

In this chapter we focus on the contribution that reflection and reflective practice can make to the development of a clinical academic career in nursing, specifically examining the use of reflective narratives and the construction of a portfolio of evidence of learning and experience.

Practice as theory generating

The shift of focus to *evidence-based practice*, such as was debated and discussed in Chapter 3, may recognize the importance of research-based nursing knowledge, but there is some doubt as to whether it sufficiently recognizes the process and experience of nursing and of nursing practice as theory generating. A shift such as this would sit more comfortably with the concepts of reflective practice and student-centered experiential learning and has the potential to offer nurse education access to an emancipatory curriculum. All this has been examined throughout this text, and as the reader will by now be aware, is inextricably linked to the process of deliberative, intentional and conscious clinical practice. One of the most pressing problems, as we have mentioned, has been that of narrowing the gap that prevails between the theory and practice of nursing.

The theory–practice gap in nursing has an established history and has been well debated, though to some extent it remains poorly understood. To reiterate some of the main arguments, Clarke (1986) highlighted three essential problems around the relationship between theory and practice:

- the separation of theory from practice
- reality versus the ideal
- nursing adherence to a scientific paradigm versus adherence to an arts paradigm.

We have addressed the above points in detail at other junctures and so will not develop the argument any further here; however, it should be noted that nurse education (and implicitly institutions of nurse education) has been heavily criticized for espousing caring ideals that do not match up to the reality of clinical practice and a number of official reports have been commissioned to explore this. It has been suggested that the theory–practice gap is one of the main causes of frustration and dissatisfaction leading to wastage of students and qualified nurses, something that many institutions struggle with constantly, and is a particular concern given the current aging population demographic globally. Some time ago Fisher *et al.* (1994: 950) categorically stated:

> *Registered nurse turnover may represent the single most serious human resource issue in health care today.*

Indeed Christine Hancock, speaking in 1999 as the General Secretary of the UK's Royal College of Nursing (RCN), informed the audience that of the many thousands of qualified nurses in the United Kingdom, a large number were not maintaining their registration. Of those that were on the register at that time only 68% were in employment. The pre-registration story is no better. Attrition rates continue to cause concern internationally, as does the recruitment of nursing students.

Every so often we read that the shortage of nurses is running at the highest level for however many years. It is maintained that the attrition rate amongst students is, therefore, no longer just an issue for academic institutions, but for the whole of nursing, not to mention the users of healthcare, namely the public. At the 1998 RCN Congress in the UK, the subject of student nurse attrition was discussed and amongst the many questions posed was: has the increasingly academic content of courses as well as a lack of understanding of the day-to-day practice of nursing contributed to and compounded the problem? (RCN, 1999: 82).

Almost 10 years later we find it interesting to read a short, anonymous editorial in the July edition of *Nursing Standard* (2006) in which concern is raised at the average figure of 25% of students leaving their courses. This is a not a new or alarmingly different statistic either nationally or globally.

In the Netherlands, the attrition rate has been known to vary between 15% and 25% per annum (Knol and de Voogd, 1990; van Rooijen, 1990), although this figure has also been quoted as varying between 25% and 40% per annum (van den Bogert, 1993). In the United States, the problem of student nurse attrition is also recognized as an area of concern to educators (Smith, 1990). This was also the case in South Africa, when in 1979 the figure was about 30% (Searle and Potgieter, 1980). More recent figures place student nurse attrition in the UK at 20% (Glossop, 2002; Last and Fulbrook, 2003). Judging from the literature, it can be assumed, therefore, that attrition is an ongoing problem and one of concern to nursing on an international scale. In the past decades this problem has been magnified due to the decreasing number of students entering initial nursing courses (Last and Fulbrook, 2003) and has possibly been compounded by the move to higher education which has excluded those students who would otherwise have entered non-degree programs.

Melia (1987), in her book *Learning and Working*, discusses the various problems facing student nurses in their development to trained nurse status. She focusses on their ability to adapt to the situations in question, and survive. There are, however, annually a great number of student nurses who do not manage this transition and who prematurely terminate their training or suffer a degree of burnout early in their nursing careers. This could partly be due the fact that Registered Nurses alter or lose their ideals, norms and values regarding their profession during their initial nursing education, or do not recognize the intrinsic motivation of novice nurses and are subsequently unable to provide them with a positive socialization to Registered Nurse status (Admi, 1997a, b; Beck and Srivastava, 1991; du Toit, 1995; Hegge *et al.*, 1999; Howkins and Ewens, 1999; Kleehammer *et al.*, 1990; Lewis *et al.*, 1987; Lindop, 1993; Policinski and Davidhizar, 1985; Siegel, 1968; Spouse, 2000; Stephens, 1992; Tanner and Raway, 1999; Tatano Beck, 1993; Tinsley and France, 2004; Wolfe Morrison, 1993).

Many years ago Allan (1989) asserted that reducing the gap between theory and practice on educational courses would assist the reduction of student wastage and the loss of registered staff, thereby improving nurse education and patient care. This seems rather naïve; whilst the theory–practice gap is of great concern to the whole of the nursing profession, it is only one of the factors influencing the attrition and retention rate in nursing. More significant factors, which also have a long history, include feeling undervalued, powerlessness and oppression within a structural hierarchy, experiencing the locus of control as external, and living with a sense of disillusionment and meaninglessness (Friedson, 1970; Johns, 1995; Roberts, 1983; Rotter, 1966; Scott, 1998).

There is little doubt that nursing and nurse education is presented with a challenge in response to these significant issues. Meeting this challenge is not simply a question of identifying where espoused theories and theories in action are in contradiction (Argyris and Schön, 1974) although evidence-based practice certainly demands that nurses maintain a closer compatibility between their caring beliefs and their nursing care. However, this is often approached by examining evidence as if it were external to the practitioner, with little attention to the body of evidence-based practice that the nurse carries around within them (Benner, 1984). This reinforces the feeling that the locus of control is external to the nurse.

It is argued that for the theory–practice gap to be addressed:

> *there has to be recognition of the interdependent and dynamic relationship between theoretical and practical knowledge. One is not superior to the other, and both are essential to improving patient care.* (Nolan *et al.*, 1998: 275)

When addressing the theory–practice gap, it is also important to make clear that it is not that nursing theory does not describe 'real nursing'; rather, it is that what is taught in the classroom is not what is practiced in the clinical situation. Attending to the theory–practice gap in the classroom by emphasizing the value of experiential knowledge *may* be one way of addressing some of the difficulties currently experienced in recruitment and retention in nursing. However, this in itself will have little effect if the nurses who bring the experiential knowledge are not also valued. In order for this to happen, a shift in locus of control is necessary, not only in the world of education and practice but also within the practitioner herself. Nurses are also required to challenge the barriers within themselves in order to recognize and own their feelings for themselves; this includes their personal power and authority.

Portfolio and narrative as emancipatory education

Portfolio development has been advocated to support professional development and there have been attempts at providing simplistic templates (Brown, 1995; Hull and Redfern, 1996). The benefit of keeping of reflective diaries or journal writing has been debated frequently in the nursing literature. Whilst it is generally seen as an advantageous learning tool, not all students respond positively and in some cases procrastination prevails (Landeen *et al.*, 1995; Paterson, 1995; Rolfe *et al.*, 2001). Structured models of reflection, such as those discussed within this text, are often used to support students in the development of writing reflectively. Students should also be encouraged to reflect in their diaries in their own writing style, whether this be semi-structured or unstructured. This is in accord with Shields (1994) who observes that:

> *Keeping a reflective journal, regardless of one's personal style, has been shown to be an effective way of evaluating experience and thus promotes learning.* (p. 755)

However, other writers assert that the aims of keeping a journal need to be clear so as to clarify the purpose both to the student and to the organization (Jasper, 2005; Lyte and Thompson, 1990). Some of the aims include:

- facilitating reconciliation of theory–practice issues through exploration of applied theory to practice;
- to assist the development of the learner's personal growth through increasing self-awareness in relation to patient and colleague interaction;
- to encourage the effective use of independent learning by stimulating motivation to set own learning objectives (Lyte and Thompson, 1990).

These aims should be made explicit to the students and incorporated into the discussion around the purpose of the reflection and portfolio development. The main purpose of a diary, however, is to stimulate learning through analysis, discussion and documentation of critical incidents/narrative events. The reflective element is confidential, but forms an important part of what might be shared and discussed in reflective process groups. It is also intended to encourage students to reflect as a regular activity.

Reflective writing is viewed as a valuable tool for the students as it has the potential to stimulate both subjectivity and objectivity, enabling students to distance themselves from an experience whilst simultaneously reporting a subjective experience (Boud *et al.*, 1993). Not only does reflective writing take the individual deeper, under their own veneer, into the domain of the psyche, but it is also a way of stepping forward and speaking their voice. Vezeau (1994: 175) confirms this stating: 'it [writing] is my most political act.' (See Chapter 8).

Furthermore, the writing and narrating of stories is closely linked to the development of consciousness through the art of reflection (Holloway and Freshwater, 2007; van Manen, 1990). Writing helps to capture events that may usually be lost in the mists of time. Reflecting on such events, the individual is able to plot their own developmental processes. In this way Burnard (1988) states the journal can be used as both an assessment and evaluation instrument. This self-assessment and evaluation process is congruent with the concept of adult education and experiential learning.

Nursing students can be asked to focus their diary on narrative events that are personally meaningful to them; these are termed critical incidents. Critical incidents have been widely used as a learning tool in general and more specifically in nurse education (Clamp, 1980; Dunn and Hamilton, 1986; Flanagan, 1954). Critical incidents are snapshot

Box 11.1 Guidelines for choosing a critical incident.

Describe a nursing incident from your clinical practice which has been significant to you because:

- you feel your intervention made a real difference to the outcome;
- the incident went unusually well;
- the incident captured the essence of nursing;
- the incident was particularly demanding;
- the incident was particularly satisfying;
- you feel the incident could have been handled differently.

In your description include details of:

- The context of the incident – where and when did it occur?
- What happened?
- Why was it significant to you?
- What were your concerns at the time?
- What were you thinking about and feeling at the time, and afterwards?
- What choices did you make, and why?
- Looking back at the incident, could you have acted in another way – what might have happened?

views of the daily work of the nurse. Used in conjunction with reflection they provide a sharply focussed lens through which opinions, personal actions, judgments and beliefs can be viewed (see Box 11.1).

The focus of the use of narrative is not the story itself but on the reader (Vezeau, 1994). This is a significant decision as nursing historically has an oral tradition (Street, 1991) and relies heavily on the reciting of stories, as can be witnessed each day at the time of the ward report. In addition, it makes appropriate space for good communication.

Discussing reflective narrative in terms of portfolio development does, however, have a different connotation for older and more experienced staff (Fuller and Unwin, 2005; Hyde and Wright, 1997). In order to respond to the changing dynamic of the healthcare or health service environment and prepare individuals for active lifelong learning, learning needs to be innovative, inclusive, relevant and flexible. There should be an approach to learning and education that will develop nurses and healthcare professionals to think analytically at an advanced level, and enable them to evaluate their practice at specialist and advanced levels. This development would be possible using an approach in which learning is experiential and work-based. Stimulating and motivating individuals to be open to learning from their experiences is, the basic premise of lifelong learning. Naturally lifelong learning could, but does not necessarily have to, be facilitated by providing a formal educational framework to which individuals bring their specific work experience in order to allow them to combine higher education with professional development using a reflective approach. Experienced staff could always utilize the principles of a work-based learning approach which include: achievement of planned learning outcomes; structured learning opportunities; learning for work and at work (Chalmers *et al.*, 2001; Clarke and Copeland, 2003) and effective interprofessional collaboration as a key factor in healthcare delivery (Prowse and Heath, 2004). The notion of learning from experience is not new and has been recognized in nursing; for example, by Benner (1984: 3) who states:

> *Expertise develops when the clinician tests and refines propositions, hypotheses, and principle-based expectations in actual practice situations. Experience is therefore a requisite for expertise.*

Incorporating work experience as a method of learning could be discussed using two approaches defined as work-related learning and work-located learning (Chapman, 2004).

In *work-related learning* the learning takes place away from work, but has the principal goal and objective of developing patient/client care in the individual's work environment. For those not directly engaged in patient/client care, the principal purpose is development of an environment/structure to allow for optimum patient/client care via a managerial/leadership, educational or research approach. The second option is *work-located learning* which involves learning at work within the individual's practice area. This is achieved through the development of accredited work-based modules. While learning is work-based and self-directed, it is also formalized by being academically accredited. Individuals clearly document their learning needs and desired outcomes, and this form of learning involves both academic and clinical supervision.

Although both approaches involve reflective skills at an advanced level, this form of learning must be placed within the context of the individual's environment. Connolly (2005: 147) referring to Lave and Wenger (1991) and Engestrom (1999) suggests that:

> *the transformative practice of a learning community offers an ideal context for developing new understandings because the community sustains the change as part of an idea of participation.*

We need to focus our attention on the individual's environment as it influences their ability to engage in reflective learning. There are a number of preconditions necessary for this type of learning to occur, as it does not occur in a vacuum, and they could be suggested as areas of reflection by experienced staff. This is an important aspect for portfolio development as it allows the individual to place their professional and personal development within the supporting and, at the same time, limiting context of their workplace.

The first precondition is the provision of personal and professional support for the individual, based on an educational philosophy. Practice is a powerful and creative learning setting in which the learner has a key role. In other words, the practitioner could reflect on their workplace's educational philosophy in terms of:

- their relationship and interaction with others;
- whether they are active and creative in their learning style;
- whether their knowledge is both rational and intuitive.

The second precondition relates to establishing a sound educational philosophy complementary to the philosophy of care on a ward or within the organization. The area of reflective journaling here would be focussed on whether these two philosophies were congruent, as the care and respect in the way a patient is approached by the nurse should be congruent to the way in which a staff member is approached as a learner.

The third precondition is the realization that learners are adults: adult learners require concrete answers to concrete questions. There should be methodic and systematic supervision in place to support the process of personal growth and development and this should tie in with the respect for the individuality of the person and focus on their search for self-actualization.

Finally, a traditional teaching and assessment method in which *punishment* becomes a negative extrinsic motivation needs to be investigated. These methods stimulate adaptation and subservient behavior and do not result in empowerment. The individual should reflect on their position in terms of power and there should be space in order to make mistakes and reflect on their process and progress. References to power and oppression have been made elsewhere in this book; by incorporating specific reflection in this area, steps could be taken towards breaking this (negative) cycle in the nursing profession.

Although experiential learning contains risks and limitations, it does link into the realistic and lived world of nurses. Being a nurse is largely

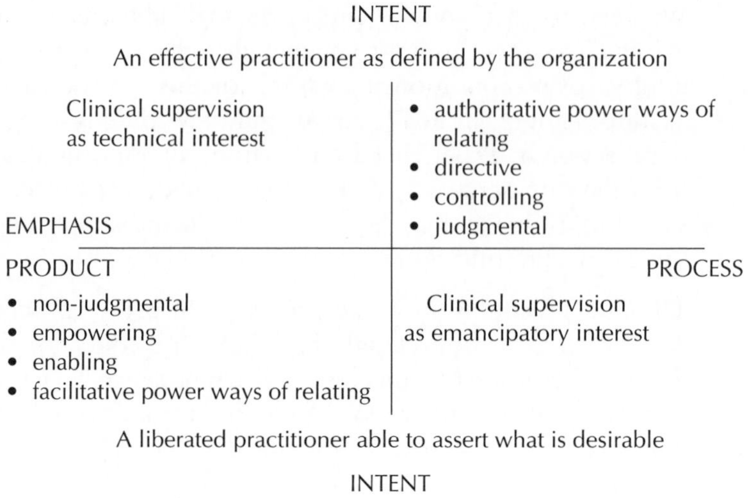

INTENT

An effective practitioner as defined by the organization

Clinical supervision
as technical interest

- authoritative power ways of
  relating
- directive
- controlling

EMPHASIS

- judgmental

PRODUCT

PROCESS

- non-judgmental
- empowering
- enabling
- facilitative power ways of relating

Clinical supervision
as emancipatory interest

A liberated practitioner able to assert what is desirable

INTENT

Figure 11.1 The intent–emphasis grid (Johns, 2001).

seen as being a practical professional, and the various types of skills needed often form the basis of competency-based education and (self-)assessment. Too little is done to develop the abstract skills nurses need – the various types of reflection, clinical decision making or communication skills. The competency-based curricula assess these outcomes, but an individual should be supported to specifically identify the intent and emphasis of their learning. The intent–emphasis grid by Johns (2001/1998) (Fig. 11.1) provides some clarity on isolating the envisaged outcomes and can be an important tool in assisting the individual in deciding whether learning as a process or a product needs to be assessed.

In their portfolio, the individual could discuss which methods of assessment they need and use as they have to contend with many variables in the course of their work. This could mean that part of their objectives is assessed in terms of outcomes, whereas other aspects would be more process-directed.

Self-directed development and work-based learning provide the individual and the organization with the potential for improving care and stimulating development. They provide nurses with a personal responsibility and allow the organization to stimulate both individual and team growth and development, ultimately leading to improved quality of care. These are important aspects for an individual when developing their career pathway, and the process of learning from work experiences allows reflection in the following areas (Esterhuizen, 2005):

- Active construction of own experience and critical reflection on the development within this experience.
- Personal identity and growth – these are central elements to the process.
- Self as part of a greater body of knowledge, and respected for their input.
- Visibility of tacit knowledge.
- Possibilities for integration of theory and practice.
- Improving the quality of care and the quality of work.
- Identification and optimal use of own potential.
- Role and cohesiveness within the healthcare team in relation to actively building and developing new insights.

These areas of reflection are vital to the individual developing their career pathway and, although the outcomes are abstract and difficult to measure, it is nevertheless important to give these outcomes a place beside the more tangible competencies healthcare professionals are being faced with (DH, 2003a, b; Skills for Health, 2003).

Development in isolation is possible and so, in deciding on the direction to be followed, journaling, portfolio development and facilitated reflection could prove to be helpful. Once decided as to the general focus of their career development – clinical, leadership, education or research – the individual will need to engage with comprehensive theoretical and practice principles towards the development of a 'practice wisdom' or 'wisdom of praxis' (Litchfield, 1999). Critical within an understanding of this process of practice wisdom are the notions of unfolding practice, transformative change, and the human role in the construction of human cultures and shared worlds. According to Litchfield (1999) recognition of the centrality of the human role in the construction of knowing and practice wisdom, or what she terms 'the creative participant,' is recognized in the scholarship of both scientist and philosopher. This is particularly pertinent within the professional practice of nursing, a discipline that is viewed as both an art and a science.

Specifically, the focus in a defined area of practice will be central to the individual's engagement with learning and reflection and, as such, it will influence both the direction of the knowledge content and the individual as a knowing professional. In other words, professional knowing will unfold in its detail, as a response to and engagement with circumstances and humanness, in context, and throughout the individual's educational experience and beyond. This is supported by Seymour *et al.* (2003: 292) who suggest that:

> *the practitioner must seek knowledge that is as unambiguous as possible and work collectively from a knowledge base that is part of a professional community.*

Thus the notion of specialist knowledge should be defined by the individual and the reflective development and application of theory and research within it, rather than by medical specialty.

This approach to learning from experience and reflecting on situations encountered in the workplace should encourage students to challenge traditional conceptualizations of quality, theory and practice. As part of their development, the individual practitioner should be open to examine and evaluate different theoretical and analytic perspectives using critical reflection on their own practice-based knowledge and patterns of knowing (Carper, 1978; White, 1995). A fundamental premise of this development is acknowledging and valuing practical knowledge; namely, assigning equal importance to the concepts of *knowing how* and formal knowledge or *knowing that.*

Part of facilitated reflection could help the individual to recognize what Spouse (1998) terms *knowledge-in-waiting* and *knowledge-in-use*, and hence, learning need. *Knowledge-in-waiting* implies learners holding a body of knowledge and a readiness to progress to the next stage, but with a limited ability to use such knowledge. In order to progress or develop their competence and expertise they need support and guidance from a more experienced colleague(s) (Spouse, 2001).

Summary

Together with the individual practitioner, the facilitator will play a pivotal role in supporting the individual to develop a learning contract (Knowles, 1990), actively embrace the notion of role modeling (Bradshaw, 1989) and participate in debriefing activities as part of reflective practice (Schön, 1988). Individuals are expected to draw upon the reality of their work-based experience to initiate and engage with the process of inquiry. Essentially three levels of knowledge should inform these processes of inquiry: knowledge-in-use, knowledge-in-waiting and evidenced-based knowing. Reflection should be broad and include empirical theories, ethical theories, personal theories and aesthetic theories within the concept of evidence-based knowing (Fawcett *et al.*, 2001). The underpinning premise to this process of learning is that the individual relates newly learned theoretical principles, evidence and skills to their practice and, in so doing, develops their expertise in practice.

References

Admi, H. (1997a) Nursing students' stress during the initial clinical experience. *Journal of Nursing Education*, 36(7), 323–7.

Admi, H. (1997b) Stress intervention: a model of stress inoculation training. *Journal of Psychosocial Nursing*, 35(8), 37–41.

Allan, P. (1989) Nursing education. A luxury or necessity? in Jolley, M. and Allen, P. (eds) *Current issues in nursing*. Chapman and Hall, London.

Argyris, C. and Schön, D.A. (1974) *Organizational Learning*. Addison-Wesley, Reading, MA.

Atkins, S. and Murphy, K. (1993) Reflection: a review of the literature. *Journal of Advanced Nursing*, 8(7), 1188–92.

Beck, D.L. and Srivastava, R. (1991) Perceived level and sources of stress in baccalaureate nursing students. *Journal of Nursing Education*, 30(3), 127–33.

Benner, P. (1984) *From Novice to Expert: Excellence and Power in Clinical Nursing Practice*. Addison-Wesley, Menlo Park, CA.

van den Bogert, E.J. (1993) Profile of first year students of higher education in nursing. A descriptive study of Dutch students. Unpublished MSDN dissertation. Hogeschool Utrecht, Netherlands.

Boud, D., Cohen, R. and Walker, D. (eds) (1993) Introduction: understanding learning from experience, in Bond, D., Cohen, R. and Walker, D. (eds) *Using experience in learning*. Oxford University Press, Oxford.

Bradshaw, P.L. (1989) *Teaching and Assessing in Clinical Nurse Practice*. Prentice Hall, Hemel Hempstead, UK.

Brown, R.A. (1995) *Portfolio Development and Profiling for Nurses*, 2nd edn. Quay Books, Salisbury, UK.

Burnard, P. (1988) The journal as an assessment and evaluation tool in nurse education. *Nurse Education Today*, 8(2), 105–7.

Carper, B.A. (1978) Fundamental patterns of knowing in nursing. *Advances in Nursing Science*, 1(1), 13–23.

Chalmers, H., Swallow, V.M. and Miller, J. (2001) Accredited work-based learning: an approach for collaboration between higher education and practice. *Nurse Education Today*, 21(8), 597–606.

Chapman, L. (2004) Practice development: advancing practice through work based learning. *Work Based Learning in Primary Care*, 2, 90–6.

Clamp, C. (1980) Learning through incidents. *Nursing Times*, 76(40), 1755–8.

Clarke, D.J. and Copeland, L. (2003) Developing nursing practice through work based learning. *Nurse Education in Practice*, 3(4), 236–44.

Clarke, M. (1986) Action and reflection: practice and theory in nursing. *Journal of Advanced Nursing*, 11(1), 3–11.

Connolly, D. (2005) Continuing professional development of occupational therapists: a case study of problem-based learning in work, in Barrett, T., Mac Labhrainn, I. and Fallon, H. (eds) *Handbook of Enquiry and Problem Based Learning*. Centre for Excellence in Learning and Teaching,

National University of Ireland, Galway, Ireland (http://www.nuigalway.ie/celt/pblbook/).

DH (Department of Health) (2003a) *The NHS Knowledge and Skills Framework (NHS KSF) and Development Review Guidance* – Working Draft (http://www.doh.gov.uk/thenhsksf).

DH (Department of Health) (2003b) *Job Evaluation Handbook*, 1st edn (http://www.doh.gov.uk/agendaforchange).

Dunn, W.R. and Hamilton, D.D. (1986) The critical incident technique: a brief guide. *Medical Teacher*, 8, 207–15.

Engestrom, Y. (1999) Activity theory and individual and social transformation, in Engestrom, Y., Miettinen, R. and Punamaki, R. (eds) *Perspectives on Activity Theory*. Cambridge University Press, Cambridge.

Esterhuizen, P. (2005) *Workshop on Work-based Learning*. Dublin: Dublin City University. Nov 28–30 2005.

Fawcett, J., Watson, J., Neuman, B., Hinton Walker, P. and Fitzpatrick, J.J. (2001) On nursing theories and evidence. *Journal of Nursing Scholarship*, 33(2), 115–19.

Fisher, M.L., Hinson, N. and Deets, C. (1994) Selected predictors of registered nurses' intent to stay. *Journal of Advanced Nursing*, 20(5), 950–7.

Flanagan, J.C. (1954) The critical incident technique. *Psychological Bulletin*, 51(4), 327–58.

Friedson, E. (1970) *Profession of Medicine*. Harper & Row, New York.

Fuller, A. and Unwin, L. (2005) Older and wiser?: workplace learning from the perspective of experienced employees. *International Journal of Lifelong Learning*, 24(1), 21–39.

Glossop, C. (2002) Student nurse attrition: use of an exit-interview procedure to determine students' leaving reasons. *Nurse Education Today*, 22, 375–86.

Hegge, M., Melcher, P. and Williams, S. (1999) Hardiness, help-seeking behavior, and social support of baccalaureate nursing students. *Journal of Nursing Education*, 38(4), 179–82.

Holloway, I. and Freshwater, D. (2007) *Narrative Research in Nursing*. Blackwell Publishing, Oxford.

Howkins, E.J. and Ewens, A. (1999) How students experience professional socialisation. *International Journal of Nursing Studies*, 36(1), 41–50.

Hull, C. and Redfern, L. (1996) *Profiles and Portfolios: A Guide for Nurses and Midwives*. Macmillan, Basingstoke, UK.

Hyde, J. and Wright, A. (1997) Self development. *Nursing Management*, 4(3), 10–11.

Jasper, M.A. (2005) Using reflective writing within research. *Journal of Research in Nursing*, 10(3), 247–60.

Johns, C. (1995) The value of reflective practice. *Journal of Clinical Nursing*, 4, 23–30.

Johns, C. (1998) *Becoming on effective practitioner through guided reflection.* Unpublished doctoral thesis, Open University.

Johns, C. (2001) Depending on the intent and emphasis of the supervisor, clinical supervision can be a different experience. *Journal of Nursing Management*, 9(3), 139–45.

Kleehammer, K., Hart, A.L. and Fogel Keck, J. (1990) Nursing students' perceptions of anxiety-producing situations in the clinical setting. *Journal of Nursing Education*, 29(4), 183–7.

Knol, H.W. and de Voogd, J. (1990) *De Uitval uit Inservice-opleidingen voor Verpleegkundigen en Zieken-verzorgenden*, Publication: 35/'90. Nationale Raad voor Volksgezondheid, Rotterdam, Netherlands.

Knowles, M.S. (1990) *The Modern Practice of Adult Education: From Pedagogy to Andragogy.* Prentice-Hall, Englewood Cliffs, NJ.

Landeen, J., Byrne, C. and Brown, B. (1995) Exploring the lived experiences of psychiatric nursing students through self-reflective journals. *Journal of Advanced Nursing*, 21(5), 878–85.

Last, L. and Fulbrook, P. (2003) Why do student nurses leave? Suggestions from a Delphi Study. *Nurse Education Today*, 23, 449–58.

Lave, J. and Wenger, E. (1991) *Situated Learning: Legitimate Peripheral Participation.* Cambridge University Press, Cambridge.

Lewis, L.L., Ford Gadd, H. and O'Conner, K. (1987) Relationship of anxiety level and recall of information to the interval between orientation and first patient care day. *Journal of Nursing Education*, 26(3), 94–8.

Lindop, E. (1993) A complementary therapy approach to the management of individual stress among student nurses. *Journal of Advanced Nursing*, 18, 1578–85.

Litchfield, M. (1999) Practice wisdom. *Advances in Nursing Science*, 22(2), 62–73.

Lyte, V.J. and Thompson, I.G. (1990) The diary as a formative teaching and learning aid incorporating means of evaluation and re-negotiation of clinical learning objectives. *Nurse Education Today*, 10(3), 228–32.

van Manen, M. (1990) *Researching Lived Experience: Human Science for an Action Sensitive Pedagogy.* State University of New York Press, Albany, NY.

Melia, K. (1987) *Learning and Working: The Occupational Socialization of Nurses.* Tavistock Publications, London.

Nolan, M., Brown, J., Naughton, M. and Nolan, J. (1998) Developing nursing's future role 2: nurses' job satisfaction and morale. *British Journal of Nursing*, 7(17), 1044–8.

Nursing Standards. July 2006. 20(43): 7. Editorial entitled Researchers look for lessons to be learned from attrition.

Paterson, B. (1995) Developing and maintaining reflection in clinical journals. *Nurse Education Today*, 15(3), 211–20.

Policinski, H. and Davidhizar, R. (1985) Mentoring the novice. *Nurse Educator*, May–June.

Powell, J.H. (1989) The reflective practitioner in nursing. *Journal of Advanced Nursing*, 14(10), 824–32.

Prowse, M.A. and Heath, V. (2004) Working collaboratively in health care contexts: the influence of bioscientific knowledge on patient outcomes. *Nurse Education Today*, 25, 132–9.

RCN (1999) *Evidence to the Review Body for 1999*. Royal College of Nursing, London.

Roberts, S.J. (1983) Oppressed group behaviour: implications for nursing. *Advances in Nursing Science*, 5, 21–30.

Rolfe, G., Freshwater, D. and Jasper, M. (2001) *Critical Reflection for Nursing and the Helping Professions: A User's Guide*. Palgrave, Basingstoke, UK.

van Rooijen, M. (1990) Werkdruk belangrijkste reden voor drop-outs. *N.M.V. visie*, 12(23/24), 13.

Rotter, J.B. (1966) Generalized expectancies for internal versus external control of reinforcement. *Psychological Monographs*, 80(609), 1–28.

Schön, D.A. (1988) *Educating the Reflective Practitioner*. Jossey Bass, San Francisco, CA.

Scott, I. (1998) Challenging the future. *Nursing Management*, 4(9), 18–21.

Searle, C. and Potgieter, E. (1980) *Nursing Education. Only Study Guide for NUE302-F*. UNISA, Pretoria, South Africa.

Seymour, B., Kinn, S. and Sutherland, N. (2003) Valuing both critical and creative thinking in clinical practice: narrowing the research–practice gap? *Journal of Advanced Nursing*, 42(3), 288–96.

Shields, E. (1994) A daily dose of reflection: developing reflective skills through journal writing. *Professional Nurse*, 9(11), 755–8.

Siegel, H. (1968) Professional socialization in two baccalaureate programs. *Nursing Research*, 17(5), 403–7.

Skills for Health (2003) *Standards database* (http://www.skillsforhealth.org.uk/standards_database/index.htm).

Smith, V.A. (1990) Student nurse attrition and implications for pre-admission advisement. *Journal of Nursing Education*, 29(5), 215–18.

Spouse, J. (1998) Learning to nurse through legitimate peripheral participation. *Nurse Education Today*, 18, 345–51.

Spouse, J. (2000) An impossible dream? Images of nursing held by pre-registration students and their effect on sustaining motivation to become nurses. *Journal of Advanced Nursing*, 32(3), 730–9.

Spouse, J. (2001) Bridging theory and practice in the supervisory relationship: a sociocultural perspective. *Journal of Advanced Nursing*, 33(4), 512–22.

Stephens, R.L. (1992) Imagery: a treatment for nursing student anxiety. *Journal of Nursing Education*, 31(7), 314–20.

Street, A. (1991) *From Image to Action: Reflection in Nursing Practice*. Deakin University Press, Geelong, Australia.

Tanner, M. and Raway, B. (1999) Socialization of the novice nursing student to the profession. *International Council of Nurses Centennial Conference*, London.

Tatano Beck, C. (1993) Nursing students' initial clinical experience: a phenomenological study. *International Journal of Nursing Studies*, 30(6), 489–97.

Tinsley, C. and France, N.E.M. (2004) The trajectory of the registered nurse's exodus from the profession: a phenomenological study of the lived experience of oppression. *International Journal for Human Caring*, 8(1), 8–12.

du Toit, D. (1995) A sociological analysis of the extent and influence of professional socialization on the development of a nursing identity among nursing students at two universities in Brisbane, Australia. *Journal of Advanced Nursing*, 21, 164–71.

Vezeau, T.M. (1994) Narrative in nursing practice and education, in Chinn, P. and Watson, J. (eds) *Arts and Aesthetic in Nursing*. National League for Nursing, New York.

White, J. (1995) Patterns of knowing: review, critique and update. *Advances in Nursing Science*, 17(4), 73–86.

Wolfe Morrison, E. (1993) Longitudinal study of the effects of information seeking on newcomer socialization. *Journal of Applied Psychology*, 78(2), 173–83.

Index